Immunotherapy and Bone Marrow Transplantation

Edited by

Thomas R. Spitzer, M.D.

Director, Bone Marrow Transplant Program
Massachusetts General Hospital
Associate Professor of Medicine
Harvard Medical School
Boston, Massachusetts

Amitabha Mazumder, M.D.

Director, Bone Marrow Transplant Program
Associate Professor of Medicine
Georgetown University School of Medicine
Washington, DC

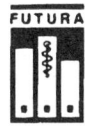

Futura Publishing Company, Inc.
Armonk, NY

Library of Congress Cataloging-in-Publication Data

Immunotherapy and bone marrow transplantation / editors, Thomas R.
   Spitzer, Amitabha Mazumder.
        p.   cm.
   Includes bibliographical references and index.
   ISBN 0-87993-602-9
   1. Bone marrow—Transplantation—Immunological aspects.
   2. Immunotherapy. I. Spitzer, Thomas R. II. Mazumder, Amitabha
   [DNLM: 1. Bone Marrow Transplantation—immunology.
   2. Immunotherapy. 3. Neoplasms—therapy.   WH 380 I33 1995]
   RD123.5.I45   1995
   617.4'4—dc20
   DNLM/DLC
   for Library of Congress   94-36234
                                                                    CIP

Copyright © 1995
Futura Publishing Company, Inc.

Published by
Futura Publishing Company, Inc.
P.O. Box 418
135 Bedford Road
Armonk, New York 10504-0418

L.C. #94-36234
ISBN #0-87993-602-9

Printed in the United States of America.

This book is printed on acid-free paper.

To our wives and children whose patience and unwavering support have allowed us to share important new information with those dedicated to the conquest of malignant disease.

Contributors

Edward D. Ball, M.D.

Chief, Division of Hematology/Bone Marrow Transplantation, Professor of Medicine, Department of Medicine, University of Pittsburgh Medical Center, Director, Bone Marrow Transplantation Program, Co-Director, Leukemia/Lymphoma Program, Pittsburgh Cancer Institute, Pittsburgh, Pennsylvania

M.J. Barnett, B.M.

Member, Leukemia/Bone Marrow Transplantation Program of British Columbia, Clinical Associate Professor, Division of Hematology, University of British Columbia, Vancouver, British Columbia, Canada

Mark C. Benyunes, M.D.

Acting Assistant Professor of Medicine, University of Washington, Associate in Clinical Research, Fred Hutchinson Cancer Research Center, Seattle, Washington

Richard Cahill, M.D.

Member, Lombardi Cancer Center, Georgetown University Hospital, Assistant Professor, Medical Oncology and Pediatrics, Georgetown University, Washington, DC, Capt., MC, U.S. Navy

Bishan S. Charak, M.D.

Research Associate, Bone Marrow Transplantation Program, Georgetown University School of Medicine, Washington, DC

Alexander Fefer, M.D.

Professor of Medicine, University of Washington, Member, Fred Hutchinson Cancer Research Center, Seattle, Washington

Allan D. Hess, Ph.D.

Bone Marrow Transplantation Program, The Johns Hopkins

Oncology Center, Professor of Oncology, Professor of Immunology and Infectious Diseases, Johns Hopkins University School of Medicine, Baltimore, Maryland

Richard J. Jones, M.D.
Director, Bone Marrow Transplantation Program, The Johns Hopkins Oncology Center, Associate Professor of Oncology, Johns Hopkins University School of Medicine, Baltimore, Maryland

Byron D. Johnson, Ph.D.
Assistant Professor, Medical College of Wisconsin, Department of Pediatrics and Cancer Center, Medical College of Wisconsin, Milwaukee, Wisconsin

Hans-G Klingemann, M.D., Ph.D.
Member, Leukemia/Bone Marrow Transplantation Program of British Columbia, Senior Scientist, Terry Fox Laboratory, British Columbia Cancer Agency, Clinical Associate Professor, Division of Hematology, University of British Columbia, Vancouver, British Columbia, Canada

T. Kühr, M.D.
Department of Medicine, University Hospital, Innsbruck, Austria

Larry W. Kwak, M.D., Ph.D.
Senior Investigator, Biological Response Modifiers Program Division of Cancer Treatment, National Cancer Institute, Frederick, Maryland

Amitabha Mazumder, M.D.
Director, Bone Marrow Transplantation Program, Associate Professor of Medicine, Georgetown University School of Medicine, Washington, DC

David H. Sachs, M.D.
Director, Transplantation Biology Research Center, Massachusetts General Hospital, Paul S. Russell/Warner-Lambert Professor of Surgery, Harvard Medical School, Boston, Massachusetts

Kathy J. Selvaggi, M.D.
Hematology/Oncology Director, Richard G. Laube Cancer Center Armstrong County Memorial Hospital, Clinical

Assistant Professor, Division of Hematology/Bone Marrow Transplantation, University of Pittsburgh, Kittanning, Pennsylvania

Megan Sykes, M.D.

Associate Immunologist, Transplantation Biology Research Center Departments of Surgery and Medicine, Massachusetts General Hospital, Associate Professor of Surgery and Medicine (Immunology) Harvard Medical School, Boston, Massachusetts

Robert L. Truitt, Ph.D.

Professor, Medical College of Wisconsin, Department of Pediatrics and Cancer Center, Medical College of Wisconsin, Milwaukee, Wisconsin

Udit N. Verma, M.D.

Research Associate, Bone Marrow Transplantation Program, Georgetown University School of Medicine, Washington, DC

Preface

Because it involves the transplantation of an immunocompetent tissue, bone marrow transplantation presents unique challenges and opportunities to both clinicians and basic immunobiologists. This book represents a state-of-the-art tribute to the fertile interactions which these challenges and opportunities have fostered.

In addition to the usual rejection response (host-versus-graft) which it has in common with all other tissue transplants, the bone marrow graft also has potential to attack the host (graft-versus-host), with the potential for causing serious disease. The practical consequences of this bi-directional activity are clear to the clinician, whose treatment must be geared toward appropriate control of both rejection and GVHD (graft-versus-host disease). The theoretical implications are equally challenging, since the entire immune system is dependent on progeny of the transplanted bone marrow and appropriate interactions with host tissues.

The implications which transplantation of bone marrow has for immunocompetent interactions in the immune system have led to wide-ranging studies of bone marrow transplantation by basic immunologists. Transplants have been used to determine how the immune system develops, especially the interactions which lead to maturation and specificity of T cells. The use of syngeneic or MHC (major histocompatibility complex)-matched bone marrow transplants has been applied to understanding the development of restriction specificity in the thymus, as well as the mechanisms of positive and negative selection leading to the peripheral T-cell repertoire. Defects apparent when differences at the MHC are imposed by mismatched transplants have been critical in determining how central and peripheral mechanisms of tolerance are regulated. These studies have also had important implications for understanding the development of autoimmunity. Finally, since bone marrow has special advantages in terms of genetic manipulation in vitro, the field of genetic engineering has required increased efforts toward understanding and controlling bone marrow stem cell development.

In this volume, the editors have assembled a series of articles which concentrate on the application of modern immunological concepts to preclinical and clinical immunotherapy and bone marrow transplantation. Topics such as autologous GVHD and cytokine interactions are covered both from a basic immunobiology point of view and with regard to potential impact on the treatment of leukemia. Indeed, all the chapters demonstrate both directly and indirectly the impact which an understanding of immunological mechanisms has had on the clinical practice of bone marrow transplantation.

David H. Sachs, M.D.
Director, Transplantation Biology
Research Center
Massachusetts General Hospital
Paul S. Russell/Warner-Lambert
Professor of Surgery
Harvard Medical School, Boston,
Massachusetts

Acknowledgments

The Editors wish to thank Virginia Enbody for her expert secretarial assistance in preparation of this book.

Contents

Chapter 1

Graft-Versus-Host Disease and the Graft-Versus-Leukemia Effect:
Lessons from Allogeneic Bone Marrow Transplantation

Robert L. Truitt, Ph.D., Bryon D. Johnson, Ph.D.

Allogeneic Bone Marrow Transplantation as a Treatment for Leukemia

The potential for using allogeneic bone marrow transplantation (BMT) as a treatment for leukemia was recognized during the ear-

This work was supported by USPHS grant CA-39854 from the National Cancer Institute, by a grant from the Midwest Athletes Against Childhood Cancer (MACC) Fund (Milwaukee, WI), and by the Cancer Center of the Medical College of Wisconsin.

liest days of experimental BMT.[1] However, the use of allogeneic bone marrow (BM) resulted in a severe and usually fatal syndrome known as "secondary disease" (to distinguish it from the "primary" disease—radiation sickness).[2] As knowledge about immune effector cells and histocompatibility antigens (HAs) evolved, it became clear that secondary disease resulted from the reactivity of immunocompetent donor cells to HAs of the host, ie, graft-versus-host (GVH) reactivity. With the development of tissue typing techniques to minimize histoincompatibility between donor and host, successful allogeneic BMT became a clinical reality, not only for the treatment of leukemia, but for a number of lethal hematologic dyscrasias.

Approximately 75% of all allogeneic BMTs are done as a treatment for leukemias and lymphomas that are largely incurable with conventional chemoradiotherapy.[3,4] Initially, the eradication of leukemia after clinical BMT was attributed primarily to the effects of high dose chemotherapy and radiation given pretransplant. However, studies in animal models and, subsequently, clinical experience in humans have shown that immunocompetent allogeneic donor cells contribute to the antileukemic effect of BMT. This immunological component is called the graft-versus-leukemia (GVL) effect.[5] The precise relationship between the beneficial antileukemia or GVL effect of allogeneic BMT and graft-versus-host disease (GVHD) remains controversial.[6,7] It has been postulated that either distinct and, therefore, separable immune effector cells are responsible for GVL and GVH reactions or that the same effector cells with differing thresholds of reactivity against leukemic and normal host cells mediate the preferential killing of leukemia.[8] In this chapter, we will briefly review general principles of GVH and GVL reactivity that are based on clinical and experimental studies of allogeneic BMT. Our goal is to provide a framework in which to understand current attempts to manipulate components of the immune system in the context of autologous BMT in order to obtain a beneficial antileukemia reaction. The focus will be on GVH/GVL reactivity after major histocompatibility complex (MHC) matched allogeneic BMT. Shown in Figure 1 is a simplified diagram of major immune effector systems that have been identified in experimental and clinical studies as contributing to the GVH syndrome.[9-12] It will be used in this chapter to discuss various GVH effector systems and their relationship to the GVL effect of allogeneic BMT.

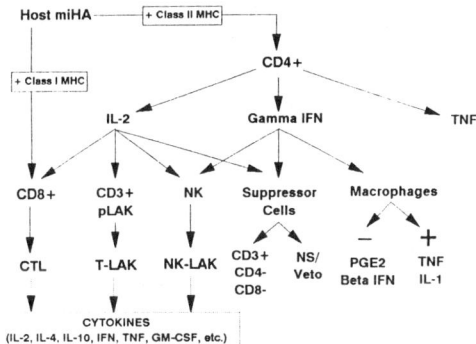

Figure 1. Simplified schema of major effector and regulatory cells and cytokines affecting GVH/GVL reactivity after MHC- matched allogeneic BMT. Alloantigen-activated donor T cells are essential for initiation of GVH reactivity. The nature (quality) and number (quantity) of activated T cells determines, in part, the incidence and severity of acute GVHD. Pleiotropic T-cell cytokines induce clonal expansion of donor T cells, recruit and activate secondary GVH effector populations, or cause direct tissue damage. In addition, these cytokines induce negative regulatory cells that may contribute to GVH-associated immune deficiency or may lead to induction of peripheral tolerance. Some secondary GVH effector cells (eg, macrophages) produce cytokines that enhance (+) and others that suppress (-) GVH reactivity. Some cytolytic effector cells (CTL, T-LAK, NK-LAK) may secrete cytokines that exacerbate the GVH reaction. Collectively, this immunological cauldron, known as the GVH syndrome, is a major determinant in the success (patient survival) or failure (patient death) of the transplant maneuver. GVHD can be influenced by prophylactic and therapeutic interventions (eg, posttransplant immunosuppression, T-cell depletion, etc.). These interventions, however, carry a risk of compromising the beneficial GVL effect associated with allogeneic BMT.

General Principles of Graft-Versus-Host Reactivity

Graft-Versus-Host Reactivity is Triggered by T-Cell Activation

The central tenets of GVH reactivity were set down by Billingham in the 1960s.[13] For a GVH reaction to occur:

1. the grafted tissue must contain immunocompetent cells;
2. the recipient must express HAs not found in the donor; and
3. the recipient must not be able to reject the transplanted cells (ie, the host must be immunoincompetent).

Small lymphocytes, later identified as mature T cells, were shown to be the immunocompetent donor cells responsible for GVH reactivity.[10] Subsequent studies established cell surface molecules encoded by the MHC (human leukocyte antigen [HLA] in man and H-2 in mouse) as the primary targets of T-cell-mediated GVH reactions[10]; however, GVH reactivity also occurred when the donor and host were matched at the MHC.[9-11] In the latter case, the targets for alloactivated T cells were presumed to be non-MHC-encoded, minor histocompatibility antigens (miHAs).[14] The crucial role for T cells in triggering GVHD across major or minor histocompatibility barriers has been well documented by pan-T cell depletion studies in both clinical and experimental settings.[15] Recent developments have forced some revision in the second of Billingham's tenets, however, in order to accommodate GVH reactions mediated by T cells that are activated inappropriately by self-antigens (ie, autoimmune reactions). Such reactions have been observed after both autologous and syngeneic BMT[16,17] and are discussed in more detail elsewhere in this volume.

If alloantigen-activated T cells persist in the host (ie, they are not rejected as stated in Billingham's third tenet), they undergo a process of differentiation and proliferation that ultimately leads to the syndrome referred to as GVHD. The immunopathologic mechanisms responsible for the GVH syndrome are complex and involve multiple populations of interacting cells and pleiotropic cytokines. Recent reviews[9-12] have summarized our current understanding of the major afferent and efferent limbs of the GVH syndrome and the role of various cytokines. The readers are directed to these sources for more details.

The Relative Contribution of CD4+ and CD8+ T Cells to Graft-Versus-Host Disease Depends on the Immunogenetic Relationship between Donor and Host

Studies with animal models have established that the immunogenetic relationship between the donor and host determines which subset of T cells is activated after BMT.[18] Cluster designation (CD)8+ T cells are activated primarily by allogeneic Class I MHC molecules, while CD4+ T cells are stimulated by allogeneic Class II MHC molecules.[19] Functional differentiation of the activated T cells correlates with the class of MHC molecule recognized: CD4+ T cells generally differentiate into cytokine-secreting T-helper cells, while CD8+ T cells differentiate into cytotoxic T lymphocytes (CTLs) or suppressor cells, but many exceptions have been noted.[18-20] Following MHC-matched BMT, similar but less well understood immunogenetic factors dictate the relative contribution of CD4+ and CD8+ T cells to the pathogenesis of GVHD.[18,19,21-23] The presumptive targets, miHAs, are a poorly defined group of endogenous self-peptides derived from a variety of cellular proteins and occupying the antigen-binding site of self-MHC molecules. Historically, miHAs have been defined by their ability to elicit allograft rejection or GVHD.

Korngold and associates in a series of studies[18,22,24] have delineated the relative contribution of populations of CD4+ and CD8+ T cells to miHA-specific GVHD. In mice that are identical at the MHC but mismatched at multiple miHA loci, depletion of CD8+ T cells is sufficient to reduce or prevent GVHD in some, but not all, combinations of donor and host.[22] CD4+ T cells are capable of inducing GVHD in only some strain combinations for reasons that are not clear, but which probably relate to the nature of the miHA disparity between donor and host.[22] Cytolytic CD8+ T cells are activated primarily, but not exclusively, by miHAs presented in the context of MHC Class I molecules[18,19]; CD4+ T cells recognize miHAs in association with Class II MHC molecules.[18,19]

A thorough discussion of miHAs is beyond the scope of this chapter. Readers are directed to reviews by Perreault et al.[14] and Loveland and Fischer-Lindahl[25] for more information. However, of interest to this review of miHA- specific GVH/GVL reactivity is a hypothesis advanced by Roopenian.[26] He has proposed that "classical" miHA loci, whose products induce allograft rejection and CTL generation, may actually be complex genetic units in which separate genes, defined by their ability to activate CD8+ cytolytic cells and CD4+ helper cells, are linked closely enough to give the illusion of segregating as a single genetic unit. Optimal immunological reactivity (eg, GVH or allograft rejection) may occur only when both CD4+ and CD8+ T cells are activated. Absence of one component or the other results in diminished reactivity. Roopenian further speculates that under appropriate circumstances, immune responses to environmental stimuli, including microbes and viruses, may provide the helper stimulus for expansion of CTLs against miHAs.[26] Conceivably, environmental antigens might also exacerbate the immunological (GVH) response to miHAs in the context of MHC-matched BMT. Support for such a possibility can be found in experimental and clinical studies of BMT under gnotobiotic conditions in which GVHD is diminished.[27-29] Also, viral infections, notably cytomegalovirus (CMV), can augment the recognition of alloantigens by T cells[30] increasing the risk of GVHD and marrow graft failure. On the other hand, a T-cell response to CMV-infected cells also may enhance the recognition of alloantigens on leukemia cells resulting in an increase in the GVL effect (ie, a decreased risk of leukemia relapse) mediated by CTLs or indirectly by cytokine-augmentation of non-T-effector cells (eg, natural killer/lymphokine-activated killer (NK/LAK) cells).[30,31]

Graft-Versus-Host Disease Depends on the Antigenic Specificity and Functional Properties of the Responding T-Cell Clones

From the work cited above and other studies, it appears that both CD4+ and CD8+ T cells contribute to GVHD directed against miHAs, although the precise nature of miHAs responsible for induction of GVH reactivity is not completely clear.[24,32] At a population level, CD8+ T cells are able to induce GVHD independent of CD4+ help.[24] Not surprisingly, the addition of CD4+ cells to an inoculum of CD8+ cells enhances the GVH potential against multiple miHAs disparities.[24] The mechanism by which CD8+ T cells mediate GVHD to miHAs without T-cell help is not clear. CD8+ cells may secrete interleukin (IL)-2 and drive their own proliferation in an autocrine fashion.[33] Alternatively, environmental antigens (eg, microbes and viruses) may provide a source of IL-2 as suggested by Roopenian[26] and Korngold.[24]

CD8+ CTLs have long been considered a major effector in GVHD at the population level. However, on a clonal level this may not always be the case.[8,33,34] For example, studies using T-cell receptor (TCR) β-chain transgenic mice demonstrate that T-cell alloreactivity does not necessarily correlate with GVH potential.[35] Rimm and colleagues[35] demonstrated that while lymphocytes from TCR-β-chain transgenic mice retained their ability to recognize allogeneic cells in vivo (by skin allograft rejection) and in vitro (by proliferative and cytotoxic assays), they were unable to induce GVHD in either irradiated or nonirradiated F_1 recipients. The failure to induce GVHD despite alloreactivity was attributed either to the limited ability of lymphocytes with a single transgenic TCR-β-chain to efficiently recognize allogeneic cells in vivo, or to the absence of critical αβ-TCR+ or γδ-TCR+ T-cell subsets that are important for mediation of the GVH reaction. In these transgenic mice, expression of endogenous β- and γ-genes is inhibited and T-cell abnormalities are observed.[35]

Early studies of T-cell function suggested that cytolytic activity and lymphokine secretion were reciprocally expressed in CD8[+] and CD4[+] T cells, respectively.[19] However, more recent studies clearly demonstrate that CD8[+] CTLs can synthesize a variety of lymphokines, including IL-2, IL-3, IL-4, IL-6, γ-interferon (IFN), tumor necrosis factor (TNF)-α and granulocyte macrophage-colony stimulating factor (GM-CSF),[36] and that CD4[+] T cells can be cytolytic.[19,34,37] The precise alloantigenic stimuli that induce lymphokine-secretion by cytolytic CD8[+] T cells are not known. After activation and expansion in vitro, Maraskovsky et al.[38] report that almost 90% of cytolytic CD8[+] murine T-cell clones secrete IL-3 and γ-IFN and approximately one-third secrete TNF following restimulation with immobilized anti-CD3, CD8 and lymphocyte function-associated antigen (LFA)-1 antibodies in the presence of IL-2. Messenger RNAs for IL-2, IL-3, γ-IFN, TNF-α, and GM-CSF can be detected by polymerase chain reaction (PCR) analysis, but in this study neither secretion nor transcripts for IL-4 and IL-6 were found.[38] This cytokine profile is similar to that reported for CD4[+] TH1 cells.[39] The absence of IL-4/IL- 6 secreting CD8[+] cells in some systems[38], but not others,[39] may relate to the presence or absence of accessory cells that provide cofactors necessary for activation and/or expansion of such cells.[38]

Cytokine-secreting CD8[+] T cells have been identified after activation during GVHD.[40] The functional characteristic that distinguishes CD8[+] T cells that secrete cytokines from those that do not is not clear, but it may have to do with expression of the IL-1 receptor.[41,42] It has been suggested that local secretion of cytokines such as γ-IFN by CD8[+] cytolytic T cells may be more important in antiviral immunity than direct lytic activity.[43] On a similar level, given the evidence that CTLs do not always cause GVHD, it is conceivable that local secretion of cytokines by CD8[+] T cells specific for host miHAs (eg, γ-IFN, IL-3, TNF-α, etc.) may be as or more important than direct target cell destruction to the pathology of GVHD, perhaps by inducing secondary effector mechanisms and/or up-regulating MHC antigen expression.

We have described two CD8[+] CTL clones that recognize Qa-1[b] but differ in their ability to cause a lethal GVH-like syndrome in vivo.[8] Both clones were cytolytic to normal and neoplastic target cells expressing Qa-1[b] in vitro. However, only one of the clones caused a rapid and severe TNF-like wasting syndrome in vivo.[8] The other clone had no GVH or cachectic activity even though it was cytolytic to normal and leukemia cells in vivo. Collectively, this and other reports[35,44,45] indicate that cytolytic activity alone is not always sufficient to cause GVHD, a conclusion that has important implications for the success of efforts to induce antitumor reactions after autologous BMT.

Antigen-activated T-helper cells are a major source of cytokines that affect the pathophysiology of GVHD. Jadus and Wepsic[12] have described the various cytokines associated with GVH reactivity, including IL-1, IL-2, IL-3, IL-4, IL-5, IL-6, γ-IFN, β-interferon (IFN), TNF-α, GM-CSF, and M-CSF among others. These cytokines regulate T cells, and B-cells, as well as other cells (NK, macrophages, hematopoietic stem cells, etc.), and some are capable of direct tissue damage. Many cytokines are pleiotropic, and the specific mechanism by which they cause GVH-associated tissue damage is not known. There is some evidence in man that the presence of proliferating, noncytolytic T cells specific for host miHAs, rather than CTLs, correlates with the incidence of severe acute GVHD.[44,45]

In an analysis of GVH mortality induced by noncytolytic CD4+ T-cell clones specific for miHAs, Miconnet et al.[46] found a clear correlation between the capacity of CD4+ clones to induce GVH mortality, to mediate delayed-type hypersensitivity (DTH), and to release high levels of TNF. They concluded that GVH mortality induced by CD4+ CD8- T-cell clones resulted from an inflammatory process associated with TNF production. Pritchard and colleagues[47] observed that CD4+ CD8- T cells mediated DTH to miHAs during a lethal GVH reaction and that the activity of these cells was regulated by CD4- CD8- ("double negative") CD3+ Thy1+ T-suppressor cells. These and other experimental data suggest that cytokines, such as TNF, act alone or in synergy with other cytokines to cause the histopathologic lesions associated with miHA-specific GVHD. As noted by Miconnet et al.,[46] this does not exclude other mechanisms, such as cytolytic T cells, in the pathology of GVHD.

Inflammatory Processes and Non-T Cells Contribute to Graft Versus Host Disease

While T cells constitute the major source of cytokines, they are neither the only source of these soluble mediators, nor the only cells that contribute to the pathophysiological effects of GVHD.[9,12] Other cells contribute through direct or indirect damage to host tissues, or by modulating immunological reactivity. For example, macrophages, activated by T-cell lymphokines such as γ-IFN or by "inflammatory mediators" such as IL-6 and IL-8, secrete a variety of factors that affect hemostasis and immunological reactivity. These include, among others, IL-1,[48] TNF,[49] β-IFN,[50] prostaglandin E_2 (PGE$_2$),[51] and various eicosanoids.[52] βIFN and PGE_2 down-regulate immunological re-activity and contribute to the profound immunosuppression associated with GVHD. Secretion of such factors represent an attempt by the body to control T cells activated after BMT.

NK cells also contribute to GVHD,[53-55] and allele-specific monoclonal antibody (MAB) directed to donor NK cells diminishes GVH-associated mortality after MHC-matched[56] and haplotype-mismatched BMT.[57] The contribution of donor NK cells to miHA-specific GVHD appears to be dependent on the presence of CD4[+] T cells.[56] Furthermore, there is no beneficial effect of NK-depletion if the number of donor T cells in the graft is high[56] or if the donor and host are fully MHC mismatched.[33,56] Thus, NK cells apparently contribute to, but are not entirely responsible for, GVHD (ie, they appear to be secondary effectors in GVHD).

Non-MHC-restricted killer cells of either T cell (CD3[+]) or NK (CD56[+] or NK1.1[+]) lineage may also contribute to the GVH syndrome. Activated natural killer (A-NK)/LAK cells secrete cytokines[58] and functionally overlap with natural suppressor/veto (NS/Veto) populations in vitro,[59] although they may be distinct in vivo.[60] NS/Veto cells are immunoregulatory cells whose precise physiological role is not known.[61,62] In animal models, they are activated by IL-2 and γ-IFN during a GVH reaction[63]; β-IFN also appears to have regulatory control over NS activity.[64] NS/Veto cells are thought to contribute to the profound immunosuppression associated with GVHD, but a role for NS/Veto cells in clinical BMT has not been established.

In summary, based on data in animal models, it appears that the capacity of CD4[+] and CD8[+] lymphocytes to provoke a lethal GVH reaction across miHA barriers depends on their antigen specificity and functional properties after activation by host-derived peptide-MHC complexes. At the clonal level, a single miHA-specific, Class I MHC-restricted CD8[+] or Class II MHC-restricted CD4[+] T-cell clone may induce lethal GVHD in vivo under appropriate experimental conditions. On a population level, it is the collective number (quantity) and nature (quality) of the responding T cells that determines the incidence and severity of GVHD. It is important to remember that host factors may also affect the GVH syndrome through an immune response directed against the graft (host-versus-graft [HVG]) or through modulation of donor immune cells via cytokine release.[65] Sykes et al.[66] have reported that one-way alloresponse to donor (HVG) as well as host (GVH) lymphohematopoietic cells could induce the state of immunosuppression that is normally attributed to GVHD. Thus, some of the efferent pathophysiological mechanisms contributing to the GVH syndrome appear to lack the immunological specificity that is responsible for their induction during afferent phases.

General Principles of Graft-Versus-Leukemia Reactivity

Evidence for a GVL effect in man is indirect and derived mostly from:

1. anecdotal reports of leukemia remission during episodes of GVHD;
2. the inverse association between GVHD and leukemia relapse found in retrospective statistical analyses of allogeneic BMT;
3. a comparison of relapse rates in recipients of marrow from monozygotic twins versus HLA-identical siblings;
4. a higher incidence of relapse following autologous BMT; and
5. the increased frequency of relapse after T-cell depletion of allogeneic donor marrow.[5]

The relative importance of an immunological component of allogeneic BMT to eradication of leukemia in humans was not fully appreciated until T-cell depletion became more widely used to prevent GVHD.[5,15] Although GVHD has been shown to be associated with an antileukemic effect, there is clinical and experimental evidence for a GVL reaction that is independent of GVHD.[5,15] Conversely, GVHD is not always accompanied by a reduction in the rate of leukemia relapse.[5,67] Despite such caveats, the GVL effect of allogeneic BMT is a dramatic example of immunological reactivity against neoplastic disease.

Although T-cell depletion has decreased the incidence and intensity of GVHD, it has not always significantly improved disease-free survival for patients with leukemia. In an analysis of patients who received T-cell-depleted BMT between 1982 and 1987, T-cell depletion was found to increase the risk of treatment failure and decrease leukemia-free survival.[15] Concern about the ultimate value of "complete" T-cell depletion in leukemia patients has led to the testing of alternate strategies in which quantitative or qualitative modifications of the T-cell content are used to decrease GVHD without the loss of the GVL effect of allogeneic BMT.[68-70] Attempts to induce GVHD in order to obtain a GVL effect in man have not always been successful.[67] On the other hand, clinical strategies designed to limit or control the GVH reaction without loss of the GVL effect have met with some success.[69,70] In the remainder of this chapter, we will review some of the general principles governing GVL reactivity in the context of MHC-matched allogeneic BMT.

There Are Multiple Graft-Versus-Leukemia Effector Cell Populations

In both humans and mice, a number of immune effector cells may act independently or in association with GVH effector cells to mediate the GVL effect (Figure 2). The relative importance of T- versus non-T-effector cells in antileukemia reactivity following allo-

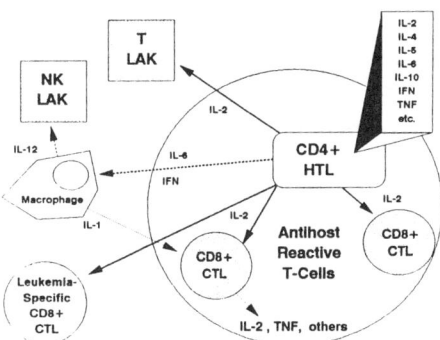

Figure 2. Relationship between GVH and GVL immune effector cell populations. Major GVL effector populations (shaded symbols) include MHC-restricted CD8+ CTL (circles) as well as MHC- unrestricted cytolytic cells of T- and NK-lineages (squares). Some GVL effector cells preferentially (or specifically) kill neoplastic host cells (shaded symbols outside large circle), while other recognize cell surface determinants, such as miHAs, expressed on both normal and neoplastic host cells (shaded symbols inside large circle). Clonal analysis indicates that some, but not all, GVL reactive CTL specific for host antigens coexpressed on leukemia cells cause severe GVHD. Cytokine secretion (possibly after costimulation with IL-1) may distinguish between GVH+ and GVH− antihost reactive CTLs. CD4+ helper T lymphocytes (HTL) secrete a variety of cytokines in response to host alloantigens. These cytokines cause direct tissue damage (tumor necrosis factor (TNF)) and/or help recruit secondary effector populations that collectively produce the GVH syndrome. GVL effector cells are dependent on CD4+ T cell derived cytokines for activation and proliferation. Pan-T-cell depletion to avoid GVHD may remove critical effector populations and/or essential cytokine-secreting HTL, leading to diminished GVL reactivity and an increased risk of leukemia relapse. The immunobiological characteristics of the host leukemia may influence which of the several GVL effector populations are operative, but other host-, donor-, and transplant-related factors, as well as posttransplant manipulations, significantly affect the reaction and clinical outcome.

geneic BMT is subject to much speculation. Studies in mice provide direct evidence for the existence of multiple GVL effector populations, but evidence for a GVL effect of T- and non-T-effector cells in man is largely indirect. Statistical analysis of data reported to the International Bone Marrow Transplant Registry (IBMTR) for patients receiving HLA-matched sibling BMT for leukemia supports the existence of three graft related antileukemia effects:

1. an antileukemia effect of GVHD;
2. an antileukemia effect of allogeneic BM grafts independent of clinically evident GVHD; and
3. an antileukemia effect that is independent of GVHD, but altered by T-cell depletion.[5]

The first two are thought to represent T-cell-mediated effects of clinical or subclinical GVHD, while the latter may represent the direct effect of T-cell-derived cytokines or activation of non-T-effector cells that do not cause GVHD, but are dependent on T cells for activation. Thus, in man, as in mice, non-T-cell GVL effectors (eg, NK/LAK cells) may be dependent on T-cell factors for their activation. High levels of A-NK/LAK cells may be necessary to compensate for the loss of GVL/GVH reactive cytotoxic T cells following T-cell depletion.[71]

We have examined the relationship between GVL reactive cytotoxic T-cell clones and GVH reactivity on a clonal level, and identified multiple GVL effector populations (Figure 2).[8,72] Some antileukemic cytotoxic T cells that are specific for miHAs cause lethal GVHD, while others do not.[8] As noted earlier, cytotoxicity alone does not correlate with ability to cause GVHD; other factors, such as ability to secrete lymphokines, appear to be critical.[8,33] Separation of antihost- and antileukemia-reactive cytotoxic cells has also been described in man, using in vitro lytic assays.[73-76] Establishing their importance to either GVL or GVH reactivity in vivo is problematic. Our studies in the AKR mouse model have shown that both CD4[+] and CD8[+] T cells are important to the GVL effect.[77,78] While both CD4[+] and CD8[+] T cells play a role, CD8[+] T cells appear to be proximal T-cell-mediators of the GVL reaction in our model[8,69] (R. Truitt, unpublished data) as well as that of others.[6,79,80] Under experimental conditions, cloned CD8[+] CTLs can mediate a GVL effect in vivo in the absence of CD4[+] T cells or exogenous growth factors.[8,33] CD4[+] T cells appear to enhance the GVL reaction primarily by inducing clonal expansion of CD8[+] T cells through secretion of IL-2. This results in a decrease in the threshold or minimum number of T cells required to achieve a curative GVL reaction.

NK cells are thought to play an important role in the development and control of hematological malignancies through "immune surveillance" mechanisms.[81] Although precursors of IL-2-activated killer cells are derived primarily from large granular lymphocytes of the NK lineage, activated MHC-unrestricted killer cells of both T (CD3[+]) and NK (CD56[+]) lineages may participate in the antitumor effect after allogeneic BMT. Precursor and fully activated LAK cells have been isolated from the peripheral blood following autologous or allogeneic BMT.[82,83] The antitumor effect of LAK cells may be mediated by direct lytic activity, as well as by the release of lymphokines such as IL-2, TNF, and γ-IFN, which act directly or indirectly on the tumor cells.[84] LAK cells have been used to restore GVL reactivity to T-cell-deficient allogeneic BM in animals,[8] and Slavin and associates[85] have shown that the GVL effect of T-cell-depleted allogeneic BMT can be enhanced by infusion of IL-2. Such studies demonstrate that exogenous non-T- effector cells and/or their cytokines can be used even in the setting of allogeneic BMT to augment GVL reactivity, bypassing the need for alloreactive T cells.

Antigen Specificity and Functional Properties of Responding Cells Determine Whether the Graft-Versus-Leukemia Effect is Separable from Graft-Versus-Host Disease

For a GVL reaction to be leukemia-specific in the truest sense of the term, the leukemia cells must express a unique antigen(s) that is not found on host cells and is presented to and recognized by immune effector cells. There are some candidate antigens (*bcr-abl*, mutated *ras*, immunoglobulin (Ig) idiotype, etc. as discussed in the next section), and leukemia-specific CTL clones have been identified.[76,86] Whether such leukemia-specific T cells are the essential GVL effectors after allogeneic BMT is difficult to prove. Indirect clinical evidence for their importance can be found in Philadelphia chromosome (Ph[1]) positive chronic myeloid leukemia (CML) where donor T cells appear to play a critical role in reducing the relapse rate posttransplant.[5] The disappearance of Ph[1+] cells after stoppage of cyclosporine in CML patients who relapse posttransplant,[87,88] remissions following the use of donor leukocyte infusions,[89,90] and emergence of CTLs reacting to host leukemia cells posttransplant[91] are all consistent with the possibility that leukemia-specific effector cells exist. If they do, then current biotechnology might allow such leukemia-specific cells to be cloned and expanded for infusion into patients. The process would be analogous to clinical trials with tumor infiltrating lymphocytes[92] and virus-specific CTLs.[93] Such strategies have been known to work in experimental models and some clinical trials (reviewed in DeVita et al.[92]).

Whether leukemia-specific T cells are induced in every transplant patient is questionable given the biological heterogeneity of their tumors. On the other hand, effector cells that recognize major or minor histocompatibility or tissue-specific antigens on leukemia cells are likely to be induced. Given the tissue distribution and differential expression of miHAs on human immunohematopoietic cells, as well as functional diversity of the allogeneic T cells that recognize them, these cells are likely to represent a major effector system in the GVL reaction.

Some miHAs appear to elicit strong GVH reactivity by activating both CD4+ and CD8+ T cells as well as secondary GVH mediators. This preferential activation of helper as well as cytotoxic T cells might account for the "immunodominance" of certain miHAs.[94] The existence of separate miHA genes or epitopes that activate either CD4+ or CD8+ T cells raises the possibility that a CD8+ CTL-mediated antileukemia reaction directed against miHA(s) could occur without an induction of the GVH-associated cytokines produced by CD4+ T cells. That is to say, preferential activation of T-cell subsets that kill leukemia cells, but not those that induce secondary immunopathological mechanisms in the GVH syndrome, could result in a GVL effect in the absence of clinically evident GVHD. Conversely, failure of miHAs to activate T-helper cells might limit the immunological potency of the cytolytic response, resulting in the progression of residual leukemia cells and relapse. Clearly, our ignorance about the biology of miHAs limits our ability to understand and predict GVH reactivity after allogeneic BMT, and to relate miHA-specific T-cell reactivity to the GVL effect. The important question may not be whether miHA-specific GVL effector cells exist, but what functional property distinguishes those that do or do not induce GVHD.

As noted earlier, some, but not all donor CTL clones specific for HAs expressed by both normal and neoplastic host cells, can provide a GVL effect in vivo without causing GVHD.[8] In addition, we have found that the lethal GVH component can be significantly reduced by selective depletion of donor CD4+ cells or NK1.1+ cells without loss of the GVL effect (see Johnson, Truitt[56] and unpublished results). In contrast, depletion of donor CD8+ T cells significantly reduces the GVL reaction, but has a less profound effect on GVH reactivity.[56,78] Optimal GVL reactivity is dependent on the presence of both CD4+ and CD8+ T cells, but not donor NK1.1+ cells.[56] The severity of GVH reactivity correlates with the CD4[+] T-cell content of the graft, not the CD8[+] content (R. Truitt, unpublished data). In the absence of CD4[+] T-helper cells, more CD8[+] T cells are required to eliminate the leukemia. In addition, efficacy of the GVL effect is influenced by the tumor load. Nevertheless, these results demonstrate that it is possible to manipulate the GVH reaction to obtain a therapeutically effective GVL reaction after MHC-matched allogeneic BMT without unacceptable GVHD.

NK and LAK effectors kill leukemia cells in vitro and may contribute to the GVL reaction in vivo.[8,84,95] Whether leukemia-killing NK/LAK cells or a subset are involved in GVHD is not clear. NK cells are among the earliest cells to emerge posttransplant,[96] and NK/LAK cells derived from BMT patients secrete a variety of cytokines,[58] many of which are associated with GVHD.[12] Experimental data indicates that depletion of donor NK1.1[+] cells results in a decrease in GVH-associated mortality without loss of GVL reactivity when T cells are present.[56] NK/LAK cells may play a more important role in the GVL effect when T cells have been removed or during the earliest days after BMT (R. Truitt, unpublished data). Preservation of MHC-unrestricted NK/LAK activity following ex vivo T-cell depletion with a MAB specific for the $\alpha\beta$-TCR-CD3 complex (T10B9) may be responsible for the low leukemia relapse rate (GVL effect) in the absence of significant acute GVHD in our clinical studies of unrelated donor BMT.[70,97] In contrast, use of CAMPATH-1, a MAB which depletes NK/LAK activity in addition to T cells,[6,98] has been associated with a low incidence of acute GVHD, but a high incidence of leukemia relapse posttransplant.[99] It should be noted, however, that there are also quantitative differences in the extent of T-cell depletion with these antibodies[98] and comparative clinical trials have not been done.

$\gamma\delta$-TCR[+] T cells represent another potential GVL effector cell population. These cells mediate MHC-unrestricted killing of leukemia and other tumor cells,[100,101] but they specifically recognize mycobacterial and other antigens in a Class I MHC-restricted manner.[102-104] They release a variety of cytokines after activation, including IL-2, IL-3, IL-4, IL-5, GM-CSF, TNF and γ-IFN.[105,106] Viale et al.[107] found that the relative percentage and absolute number of $\gamma\delta$[+] cells among CD3[+] T lymphocytes was high in marrow transplanted patients, especially in those presenting with acute GVHD. It is worth noting that $\gamma\delta$[+] T cells are spared by the $\alpha\beta$-TCR-CD3-specific T10B9 antibody (Carolyn Keever, personal communication) used successfully to reduce acute GVHD without loss of the GVL effect in the BMT program at our institution.[70] Direct evidence for a GVL role of $\gamma\delta$[+] T cells, however, is lacking.

Immunological Characteristics of Leukemia Affect Susceptibility to Graft-Versus-Leukemia Effector Cells

As a general rule, spontaneously arising tumors in man and animals tend to be poorly immunogenic in an autochthonous or a syngeneic host. As a consequence, tumor-specific MHC-restricted helper or cytolytic T cells may not be activated in sufficient numbers to benefit the tumor-bearing host. There are, however, unique tumor-associated antigens that elicit such reactivity.[108] Novel fusion proteins, such as those produced by the *bcr-abl* translocation in CML[109] may serve as leukemia-specific antigens for T cells. Mutations in the *ras* protein, commonly detected in several human tumors, produce new epitopes that can be recognized as tumor-specific proteins by T cells.[110] Ig idiotypes expressed on leukemia cells of B-cell origin represent another unique type of leukemia-specific antigen capable of eliciting a therapeutic immune response.[111] In animal models, retrovirus-associated glycoproteins are potential targets of T-cell-mediated GVL reactivity, and leukemia-specific T cells have been described in syngeneic animal models.[112,113]

Although leukemia-specific T cells have been shown to exist in some clinical and experimental studies, their role in de novo GVL reactivity following allogeneic BMT is unclear. Few experimental or clinical studies have examined leukemia-specific T cells in the setting of allogeneic BMT[72,75,86,114] where detection of tumor-specific reactivity is confounded by alloreactivity. While one cannot exclude the possibility that GVL reactivity may be directed against unique leukemia-associated antigens, it is much more likely that normal HAs expressed on allogeneic leukemia cells are the principal targets for GVL effector cells after allogeneic BMT. In the absence of any leukemia-specific antigens, GVL reactivity mediated by donor-derived MHC-restricted T cells would be limited to recognition of host alloantigens (MHC, miHA, leukocyte differentiation antigens, etc.). As a result, the extent of genetic disparity between donor and host (as well as the T-cell content of the graft) would dictate the potency of the GVL reaction and its relationship to GVHD. With increasing genetic identity, the number of potential alloantigenic targets for GVL reactivity would be reduced until the T-cell component contributes little or nothing to eradication of the leukemia. Furthermore, since antigen-activated T cells are essential for initiation of the cytokine cascade, secondary GVL/GVH effector systems (eg, MHC-unrestricted T cells, NK/LAK cells, etc.) may also be compromised. This may account for the high relapse rates observed after transplantation of BM between monozygotic twins.[115] The nature of the miHA on leukemia cells (ie, whether they activate either CD4⁺ or CD8⁺ T cells, or both) may also influence the GVL reactivity in a given donor-host pair as noted in the earlier discussion on GVHD.

Intercellular cell adhesion molecules (CAM) are critical to efficient cellular recognition by antigen-specific TCR⁺ T cells, as well as by effector cells that lack TCRs (eg, CD3⁻ MHC-unrestricted LAK cells). Initial contact between a CTL and its target cell, for example, involves receptor-ligand binding between LFA-1 and ICAM-1 [116,117]. This low affinity binding facilitates recognition of the peptide-MHC complex on the target cell by the αβ-TCR-CD3 complex of the CTL and efficient delivery of cytotoxic molecules (ie, killing of the target). In the absence of antigen recognition, the CTL detaches from the target cell without killing it. Other receptor-ligand interactions mediate effector-target cell contact using similar mechanisms (eg, CD2 and LFA-3/CD58; CD11a/CD18 and CD54). NK and LAK cells, which may be CD3⁺ or CD3⁻,[118,119] also require adhesion molecules for efficient binding and killing of target cells.[120,121] Oblakowski et al.[121] suggest that the preferential lysis of malignant CD34⁺ myeloid cells over normal CD34⁺ myeloid cells by LAK cells is due to differential expression of the CD54 ligand that interacts with CD11a/CD18 (LFA-1) receptor on either CD2⁺ or CD2⁻ LAK cells.

Tumor cells are known to vary in their expression of MHC molecules and CAMs. Limited or absent expression of certain CAMs, peptide-presenting MHC molecules, or other accessory molecules essential for target recognition and/or signal transduction, may diminish or obviate the ability of effector cells to recognize and kill leukemia cells. As a result, even if MHC-restricted or MHC-unrestricted immune effector cells are present posttransplant, the leukemia itself, by virtue of its immunological characteristics, can influence whether or not a GVL reaction occurs. In the absence of any appropriate CAMs, the leukemia cells may escape immunological destruction even when the patient experiences severe GVHD. On the other hand, CAMs are up- regulated by various cytokines.[122] Thus,in the recipient of an allogeneic BMT, T-cell-derived cytokines may activate effector mechanisms and enhance the susceptibility of the leukemia cells to kill, resulting in a preferential GVL effect (with or without clinically evident GVHD).

Graft-Versus-Leukemia/Graft-Versus-Host Effector Cells are Subject to Immunoregulatory Control

For leukemic hosts, it is critical that we fully understand how various factors impact on the elimination of leukemia in order to develop a rationale for clinical strategies to achieve long-term disease-free survival. In analyzing the results of T-cell-depleted marrow allografts reported to the IBMTR, Marmont et al.[15] identified a number of controllable factors that influenced the success of such transplants, including: the dose; dose rate and fractionation of total body irradiation (TBI) used to condition the host; the type of post-transplant immunosuppression (ie, whether cyclosporin was used); and the method of T-cell depletion. We have used a murine model to explore the relationships between some of these factors (ie, pre-transplant conditioning, T-cell and T-subset depletion of donor cells) with regard to GVHD and T-cell chimerism, and to determine how chimerism and GVHD affect GVL reactivity.[77,78] The results demonstrate that both the pretransplant conditioning regimen and the dose of alloreactive T cells in the marrow inoculum affect the extent of donor T-cell chimerism and, consequently, the severity of GVHD. Complete donor T-cell engraftment is necessary for an effective GVL reaction, but also results in an increased risk of GVHD. When host mice are conditioned for transplantation with suboptimal TBI, so that competitive host immunohematopoietic stem cells persist, donor T cells (especially CD8+ T cells) are essential for achieving complete engraftment by eliminating residual host cells. In the model used, transplantation of MHC-matched donor BM without T cells results in mixed chimerism, whereas mice given BM with T cells develop into complete and stable donor chimeras.[77] Depletion of T-cell subsets is associated with a marked increase in the frequency of mixed T-cell chimerism and loss of GVL reactivity [78]. Mixed chimerism has been described after allogeneic BMT in man,[123-125] but its effect on GVL reactivity is not clear. Using sensitive molecular techniques together with cytogenetic analysis, Lawler et al.[125] report that the proportion of patients with mixed donor-host chimerism can exceed 80% after T-cell-depleted BMT. While mixed chimerism is not a direct indicator of relapse, patients with mixed chimerism have a less favorable outcome.[125] The persistence of host cells after allogeneic BMT suggests that the immunohematopoietic environment might also tolerate the presence of residual leukemia cells.

Resolution of GVHD depends in part on the development of immunological tolerance between the donor and host. While tolerance to self MHC molecules is thought to be the result of clonal deletion of autoreactive immature lymphocytes in the thymus,[126] extrathymic tolerance can also develop through mechanisms such as suppression[127,128] and clonal anergy.[129] Theoretically, the development of donor-host-tolerance has potential for increasing the risk of relapse by allowing leukemia cells to persist. In an animal model, tolerance can prevent GVL reactivity in a time dependent manner.[130] That is, the ability of animals undergoing clinical GVHD to mount a therapeutically effective GVL reaction diminishes with time. If immunological tolerance between donor and host is achieved before any residual leukemia is eliminated, then the risk of relapse will increase. The factors that determine when and whether donor-host-tolerance develops after allogeneic BMT in man are unknown; however, animal studies suggest that T-cell depletion may accelerate the development of tolerance or suppressor-inducing systems.[78,130] Studies in mice[131] (B.D. Johnson, unpublished data) show that the predominant population of T cells in the thymus during the first two weeks after marrow transplantation are host-derived; whereas, those present at later times are derived from the donor. Mature donor-derived T cells emigrating from the thymus of the marrow recipient may be tolerant of the MHC-matched host as a result of negative selection in the thymus, extrathymic suppressor mechanisms, or both. Eradication of leukemia may depend on the strength and speed of the GVL/GVH reactions in relation to the rate at which tolerance develops.

The mechanism or mechanisms of tolerance to miHAs in the context of MHC-compatible BMT are not well defined, and the consequence of donor-host-tolerance in human BMT is unknown. Perreault et al.[132,133] examined donor-host-tolerance in a murine model of MHC-compatible BMT. Although suppressor cells were thought to establish and maintain tolerance, they could not identify natural suppressor cells, veto cells or anti-idiotypic T-suppressor cells as the responsible cell type.[133] These investigators did demonstrate, however, that the number of donor T cells administered to the host determined whether GVHD or tolerance developed after MHC-compatible BMT.[132]

The importance of donor cells in maintaining a remission after transplantation for CML has been emphasized in BMT patients who relapsed several years after receiving one or more HLA-identical sibling marrow grafts for CML.[89,90] While α-IFN therapy failed to induce a remission, repeated infusions of donor leukocytes induced complete cytogenetic and hematologic remissions. None of the patients had developed severe GVHD prior to relapse, but some developed mild GVHD after infusion of leukocytes. Host-type hematopoietic cells disappeared after the infusions, and the patients remained in complete remission for as long as they had been followed (up to 91 weeks after treatment).

These anecdotal reports lend support to the hypothesis that some leukemia relapses post-BMT are the result of a suboptimal

GVL/GVH reaction. The suboptimal response could be due to development of donor-host-tolerance or suppression of the GVH reaction before elimination of the leukemic clone. Alternatively, they could be due to an insufficient number of alloreactive, mature T cells in the graft. In either case, infusion of immunocompetent lymphocytes obtained from the donor successfully induced an apparent GVL reaction with or without clinical GVHD. It should be kept in mind, however, that if the donor-host pair is matched at MHC and non-MHC loci to such an extent that alloreactivity does not occur, or if the leukemia cells lack appropriate target molecules, then infusion of T-cell-rich mononuclear cell suspensions might not increase the frequency of GVL/GVH effector cells.

Induction of tolerance to the host is not always accompanied by loss of GVL reactivity. For example, Sykes and colleagues[80,134,135] have demonstrated in a fully MHC-mismatched BMT mouse model that administration of a short course of high dose IL-2 (with or without coadministration of T-cell-depleted host marrow) diminishes GVHD without compromising the GVL effect. The mechanism by which GVL and GVH reactivity were dissociated appears to be the selective inhibition by IL-2 of the GVH-production activity of donor CD4+ T cells.[80] CD8+ T cells, which mediate the GVL effect against EL4 leukemia/lymphoma in this model, did not cause GVHD and were not inhibited by IL-2 treatment even when they were obtained from donor mice presensitized to host skin grafts. The precise mechanism for selective inhibition of CD4-mediated GVHD is not known, but it occurs independently of NK cells, LAK cells or their precursors[60] or host T cells.[80] TCR+ CD4- CD8- T cells may play a role.[136]

Bortin and colleagues[137] were among the first to show that GVL reactivity could be dissociated from GVHD. They were able to induce GVL reactivity in MHC-matched allogeneic donors without an increase in GVH-associated mortality by selective alloimmunization to miHAs. The primary GVL effector cells in this model were later identified as CD8+ T cells primed to host miHAs,[8,72,138] but the precise mechanism by which GVL reactivity was selectively augmented without an increase GVHD was not identified. Studies by Halle-Pannenko and colleagues,[139-141] however, shed some light on the mechanism. In a series of studies, they have established that sensitization or alloimmunization of the donor to host miHAs induces a population of double negative (CD3+ CD4- CD8-) T-suppressor cells which abrogate miHA-specific DTH and GVH-associated mortality attributed to CD4+ T cells.[140] A similar alloimmunization-induced suppressor-mediated mechanism may account for the preferential GVL effect (mediated by CD8+ T cells) without exacerbation of GVHD (induced by CD4+ T cells) as described by Bortin et al.[137]

The independent models developed by Pritchard, Halle- Pannenko and colleagues,[141] Sykes et al.,[80] and Bortin et al.,[137] all suggest that GVL/GVH effector cells are under significant regulatory control. Preliminary results from studies in progress in our laboratory indicate that alloreactive CD4[+] T cells induce donor NK1.1[+] to suppress (directly or indirectly) the GVL reactivity of CD8[+] T cells.[142] Depletion of either the CD4 or the NK1.1 component allows the GVL reaction to proceed. Thus, it is possible, at least in mice, to manipulate regulatory and effector systems to avoid the GVH-component of allogeneic BMT without loss of the GVL-component.

Summary

The GVL effect of allogeneic BMT is a dramatic example of immune effector mediated antitumor reactivity. In this chapter, we have described various effector systems for GVL reactivity and their relationship to GVHD. While the GVL effect is often associated with development of GVHD, the presence of GVHD does not guarantee an antileukemic effect and the absence of clinical GVHD does not indicate the absence of an antileukemic effect. Both experimental and clinical data indicate that multiple T-cell and non-T-cell effector systems are involved in the GVL effect. Some, but not all of them contribute to the complex syndrome of GVHD.

While GVL/GVH reactivity is strongly influenced by the immunogenetic relationship of the donor to the recipient, the immunobiology of the leukemia itself also influences the reaction. Clinical strategies designed to prevent or modulate GVHD, especially T-cell depletion, increase the risk of relapse by eliminating both GVL and GVH effector cells. Mixed chimerism and donor-host-tolerance are manifestations of immunological reactivity between donor and host cells that can significantly affect relapse after BMT. Whether an effective (curative) or ineffective (relapse), reaction develops in the presence or absence of GVHD may depend, in part, on the number and nature of GVL/GVH effector and regulatory systems activated posttransplant. It is critical that we understand the various systems involved, how they interact, and how they are affected by pretransplant and posttransplant interventions if we are to improve long-term disease-free survival in patients with hematologic malignancies. Only a thorough understanding of GVL and GVH effector systems and their regulation in the setting of allogeneic BMT will allow us to design clinical protocols to manipulate these reactions for the benefit of leukemia patients, and possibly adapt them to autologous settings.

References

1. Barnes DWH, Corp MJ, Loutit JF, et al: Treatment of murine leukemia with X-rays and homologous bone marrow. Br Med J 2:626-627, 1956.
2. van Bekkum DW, de Vries MJ: Radiation Chimeras. London, Logos Press, 1967.
3. Bortin MM, Rimm AA: Increasing utilization of bone marrow transplantation. Transplantation 42:229-234, 1986.
4. Bortin MM, Rimm AA: Increasing utilization of bone marrow transplantation. II. Results of the 1985-1987 survey. Transplantation 48:453-458, 1989.
5. Horowitz MM, Gale RP, Sondel PM, et al: Graft-versus-leukemia reactions after bone marrow transplantation. Blood 75:555-562, 1990.
6. Slavin S, Ackerstein A, Naparstek E, et al: The graft-versus-leukemia (GVL) phenomenon: Is GVL separable from GVHD? Bone Marrow Transplant 6:155-161, 1990.
7. Gale RP, Champlin RE: How does bone-marrow transplantation cure leukaemia? Lancet 2(8393):28-30, 1984.
8. Truitt RL, LeFever AV, Shih CY, et al: Graft-versus-leukemia effect. In SJ Burakoff, HJ Deeg, J Ferrara, K Atkinson (eds): Graft-vs-Host Disease: Immunology, Pathophysiology, and Treatment. New York, NY, Marcel Dekker, 1990, pp 177-204.
9. Burakoff SJ, Deeg HJ, Ferrara J, Atkinson K: Graft-vs-Host Disease: Immunology, Pathophysiology, and Treatment. New York, NY, Marcel Dekker, 1990.
10. Ferrara JLM, Deeg HJ: Graft-versus-host disease. N Engl J Med 324:669-674, 1991.
11. Parkman R: Graft-versus-host disease. Annu Rev Med 42:189-197, 1991.
12. Jadus MR, Wepsic HT: The role of cytokines in graft-versus-host reactions and disease. Bone Marrow Transplant 10:1-14, 1992.
13. Billingham RE: The biology of graft-versus-host reactions. Harvey Lect 62:21-78, 1966.
14. Perreault C, Decary F, Brochu S, et al: Minor histocompatibility antigens. Blood 76:1269-1280, 1990.
15. Marmont AM, Horowitz MM, Gale RP, et al: T-cell depletion of HLA-identical transplants in leukemia. Blood 78:2120-2130, 1991.
16. Parkman R: Graft-versus-host disease: An alternative hypothesis. Immunol Today 10:362-364, 1989.

17. Bos GMJ, Majoor GD, van Breda Vriesman PJC: Graft-versus-host disease: The need for a new terminology. Immunol Today 11:433-436, 1990.
18. Korngold R, Sprent J: T-cell subsets and graft-versus-host disease. Transplantation 44:335-339, 1987.
19. Sprent J, Webb SR: Function and specificity of T cell subsets in the mouse. Adv Immunol 41:39-133, 1987.
20. Mosmann TR, Schumacher JH, Street NF, et al: Diversity of cytokine synthesis and function of mouse CD4$^+$ T cells. Immunol Rev 123:209-229, 1991.
21. Parkman R: Clonal analysis of murine graft-versus-host disease: I. Phenotype and functional analysis of T lymphocyte clones. J Immunol 136:3543-3548, 1986.
22. Korngold R, Sprent J: Variable capacity of L3T4$^+$ T cells to cause lethal graft-versus-host disease across minor histocompatibility barriers in mice. J Exp Med 165:1552-1564, 1987.
23. OKunewick JP, Kochiban DL, Buffo MJ: Comparative effects of various T cell subtypes on GVHD in a murine model for MHC-matched unrelated donor transplant. Bone Marrow Transplant 5:145-152, 1990.
24. Korngold R: Lethal graft-versus-host disease in mice directed to multiple minor histocompatibility antigens: Features of CD8$^+$ and CD4$^+$ T cell responses. Bone Marrow Transplant 9:355-364, 1992.
25. Loveland BE, Fischer-Lindahl K: The definition and expression of minor histocompatibility antigens. In J McCluskey (ed): Antigen Processing and Recognition. Boca Raton, Fla, CRC Press, 1991, pp 173-192.
26. Roopenian DC: What are minor histocompatibility loci? A new look at an old question. Immunol Today 13:7-10, 1992.
27. Beelen DW, Haralambie E, Brandt H, et al: Evidence that sustained growth suppression of intestinal anaerobic bacteria reduces the risk of acute graft-versus-host disease after sibling marrow transplantation. Blood 80:2668-2676, 1992.
28. Vossen JM, Heidt PJ: Gnotobiotic measures for the prevention of acute graft-vs-host disease. In SJ Burakoff, HJ Deeg, J Ferrara, K Atkinson (eds): Graft-vs.-Host Disease: Immunology, Pathophysiology and Treatment. New York, NY, Marcel Dekker, 1990, pp 403-423.
29. Truitt RL: Application of germ free techniques to the treatment of leukemia in AKR mice by allogeneic bone marrow transplantation. In H. Waters (ed): The Handbook of Cancer Immunology. Volume 5: Immunotherapy. New York, NY, Garland STPM Press, 1978, pp 431-452.

30. Jacobsen N, Badsberg JH, Lonnqvist B, et al: Graft-versus-leukemia activity associated with CMV-seropositive donor, post- transplant CMV infection, young donor age and chronic graft-versus-host disease in bone marrow allograft recipients. Bone Marrow Transplant 5:413-418, 1990.
31. Duncombe AS, Grundy JE, Prentice HG, et al: CMV-induced augmentation of GVL effect may be mediated by cytokines. Bone Marrow Transplant 7:69, 1991. Letter.
32. Maier T, Claman HN: Experimental GVHD across minor histocompatibility barriers. In SJ Burakoff, HJ Deeg, J Ferrara, K Atkinson (eds): Graft-Versus-Host Disease: Immunology, Pathophysiology and Treatment. New York, NY, Marcel Dekker, 1990, pp 75-94.
33. Vallera DA, Blazar BR, Widmer MB: T-cell clones in graft-vs.-host disease. In SJ Burakoff, HJ Deeg, J Ferrara, K Atkinson (eds): Graft-Versus-Host Disease: Immunology, Pathophysiology, and Treatment. New York, NY, Marcel Dekker, 1990, pp 61-73.
34. Parkman R: Clonal analysis of graft-vs.-host disease. In SJ Burakoff, HJ Deeg, J Ferrara, K Atkinson (eds): Graft-vs-Host Disease: Immunology, Pathophysiology, and Treatment. New York, NY, Marcel Dekker, 1990, pp 51-60.
35. Rimm IJ, Ghayur T, Gasser DL, et al: Alloreactive lymphocytes from T cell receptor (β-chain) transgenic mice do not mediate a graft-versus-host reaction. J Immunol 146:1130-1133, 1991.
36. Kelso A, Troutt AB, Maraskovsky E, et al: Heterogeneity in lymphokine profiles of CD4+ and CD8+ T cells and clones activated in vivo and in vitro. Immunol Rev 123:85-114, 1991.
37. Shih CY, Truitt RL: Downregulation of L3T4+ cytotoxic T lymphocytes by interleukin-2. Science 238:344-347, 1987.
38. Maraskovsky E, Rogers LA, Troutt AB, et al: Murine cytolytic CD8+ T cell clones generated in a high cloning efficiency, accessory cell-free culture system express a restricted lymphokine profile. Cell Immunol 141:59-70, 1992.
39. Fong TA, Mosmann TR: Alloreactive murine CD8+ T cell clones secrete the Thl pattern of cytokines. J Immunol 144:1744-1752, 1990.
40. Kelso A: Frequency analysis of lymphokine-secreting CD4+ and CD8+ T cells activated in a graft-versus-host reaction. J Immunol 145:2167-2176, 1990.
41. Mizuochi T, McKean DJ, Singer A: IL-1 as a co-factor for lymphokine-secreting CD8+ murine T cells. J Immunol 141:1571-1575, 1988.

42. Klarnet JP, Kern DE, Dower SK, Matic LA, Cheever MA and Greenberg PD: Helper-independent CD8+ cytotoxic T lymphocytes express IL-1 receptors and require IL-1 for secretion of IL-2. J Immunol 142:2187-2191, 1989.

43. Ruby J, Ramshaw I: The antiviral activity of immune CD8+ T cells is dependent on interferon-gamma. Lymphokine Cytokine Res 10:353-358, 1991.

44. Van Els CACM, Bakker A, Zwinderman AH, et al: Effector mechanisms in graft-versus-host disease in response to minor histocompatibility antigens. I. Absence of correlation with cytotoxic effector cells. Transplantation 50:62-66, 1990.

45. Van Els CACM, Bakker A, Zwinderman AH, et al: Effector mechanisms in graft-versus-host disease in response to minor histocompatibility antigens. II. Evidence of a possible involvement of proliferative T cells. Transplantation 50:67-71, 1990.

46. Miconnet I, Huchet R, Bonardelle D, et al: Graft-versus-host mortality induced by noncytolytic CD4+ T cell clones specific for non-H-2 antigens. J Immunol 145:2123-2131, 1990.

47. Pritchard LL, Huchet R, Bruley-Rosset M, et al: Induction and suppression of delayed-type hypersensitivity to non-MHC antigens during lethal graft-versus-host reaction. J Immunol 149:45-52, 1992.

48. Gerrard TL, Siegel JP, Dyer DR, et al: Differential effects of interferon-α and interferon-γ on interleukin 1 secretion by monocytes. J Immunol 138:2535-2540, 1987.

49. Nedwin GE, Suedersky LP, Bringman TS, et al: Effect of IL-2, IFN, and mitogens on the production of tumor necrosis factors α and β. J Immunol 35:2492-2497, 1985.

50. Cleveland MD, Ramirez RB, Klimpel GR: IFN-β production by macrophages obtained from mice undergoing graft versus host disease. J Immunol 141:3823-3827, 1988.

51. Lapp WS, Mendes M, Kirchner H, et al: Prostaglandin synthesis by lymphoid tissue of mice experiencing a graft versus host reaction: Relationship to immunosuppression. Cell Immunol 50:271- 281, 1980.

52. Foegh ML, Hartmann DP, Rowles JR, et al: Leukotrienes, Thromboxane, and Platelet activating factor in organ transplantation. Adv Prostaglandin Thromboxane Leukotriene Res 17:140-146, 1987.

53. Ghayur T, Seemayer TA, Kongshavn PAL, et al: Graft-versus-host reactions in the beige mouse: An investigation of the role of host and donor natural killer cells in the pathogenesis of GVH disease. Transplantation 44:261-267, 1987.

54. Ghayur T, Seemayer TA, Lapp WS: Prevention of murine graft-versus-host disease by inducing and eliminating ASGM1⁺ cells of donor origin. Transplantation 45:586-590, 1988.
55. Ferrara JL, Guillen FJ, van Dijken PJ, et al: Evidence that large granular lymphocytes of donor origin mediate acute graft- versus-host disease. Transplantation 47:50-54, 1989.
56. Johnson BJ, Truitt RL: A decrease in graft-vs-host disease without loss of graft-vs-leukemia reactivity after MHC-matched bone marrow transplantation by selective depletion of donor NK cells in vivo. Transplantation 54:104-112, 1992.
57. MacDonald GC, Gartner JG: Prevention of acute lethal graft-versus-host disease in F_1 hybrid mice by pretreatment of the graft with anti-NK-1.1 and complement. Transplantation 54:147-151, 1992.
58. Perussia B: Lymphokine-activated killer cells, natural killer cells and cytokines. Current Opinion Immunol 3:49-55, 1991.
59. Saffran DC, Singhal SK: Further characterization of murine bone marrow-derived natural suppressor cells. Potential relationships between NS and NK/LAK activities. Cell Immunol 128:301-313, 1990.
60. Sykes M, Abraham VS: The mechanism of IL-2-mediated protection against GVHD in mice. II. Protection occurs independently of NK/LAK cells. Transplantation 53:1063-1070, 1992.
61. Schwadron RB, Palathumpat V, Strober S: Natural suppressor cells derived from adult spleen and thymus. Transplantation 48:107-110, 1989.
62. Fink PJ, Shimonkevitz RP, Bevan MJ: Veto cells. Annu Rev Immunol 6:115-137, 1988.
63. Holda JH, Maier T, Claman HN: Natural suppressor activity in graft-vs-host spleen and normal bone marrow is augmented by IL-2 and interferon-γ. J Immunol 137: 3538-3543, 1986.
64. Cleveland MG, Lane RG, Klimpel GR: Spontaneous IFN-β production. A common feature of natural suppressor systems. J Immunol 141:2043-2049, 1988.
65. Gale RP, Horowitz MM, Butturini A, et al: What determines who develops graft-versus-host disease: The graft or the host (or both)? Bone Marrow Transplant 10:99-102, 1992.
66. Sykes M, Sheard MA, Sachs DH: Graft-versus-host-related immunosuppression is induced in mixed chimeras by alloresponses against either host or donor lymphohematopoietic cells. J Exp Med 168:2391-2396, 1988.
67. Sullivan KM, Storb R, Buckner CD, et al: Graft-versus-host disease as adoptive immunotherapy in patients with advanced hematologic neoplasms. N Engl J Med 320:828-834, 1989.

68. Butturini A, Gale RP: New strategies for T cell depletion. Bone Marrow Transplant 6:225-227, 1990.
69. Champlin R, Ho W, Gajewski J, et al: Selective depletion of CD8[+] T lymphocytes for prevention of graft-versus-host disease after allogeneic bone marrow transplantation. Blood 76:418-423, 1990.
70. Ash RC, Casper JT, Chitambar CR, et al: Successful allogeneic transplantation of T-cell depleted bone marrow from closely HLA-matched unrelated donors. N Engl J Med 322:485-494, 1990.
71. Prentice HG, Brenner MK: The benefits and drawbacks of T-cell-depletion in human allogeneic bone marrow transplantation for the treatment of leukemia. In M Martelli, F Grignani, Y Reisner (eds): T-Cell-Depletion in Allogeneic Bone-Marrow Transplantation. Rome, Serono Symposia, 1988, pp 131-137.
72. Truitt RL, Shih CY, LeFever AV, et al: Characterization of alloimmunization-induced T-lymphocytes reactive against AKR leukemia in vitro and correlation with graft-versus-leukemia reactivity in vivo. J Immunol 131:2050-2058, 1983.
73. Hercend T, Takvorian T, Nowill A, et al: Characterization of NK cells with antileukemia activity following allogeneic bone marrow transplantation. Blood 67:722-728, 1986.
74. van Rood, JJ, Goulmy E, van Leeuwen A: The immunogenetics of chronic graft-vs-host disease and its relevance for the graft-vs-leukemia effect. Prog Clin Biol Res 244:433-438, 1987.
75. Sosman JA, Oettel KR, Hank JA, et al: Specific recognition of human leukemic cells by allogeneic T cell lines. Transplantation 48:486-495, 1989.
76. Sosman JA, Oettel KR, Smith SD, et al: Specific recognition of human leukemic cells by allogeneic T cells. II. Evidence for HLA-D restricted determinants on leukemic cells which are crossreactive with determinants present on unrelated non-leukemic cells. Blood 75:2005-2016, 1990.
77. Truitt RL, Atasoylu AA: Impact of pretransplant conditioning and donor T cells on chimerism, graft-vs-host disease, graft-vs-leukemia reactivity, and tolerance after bone marrow transplantation. Blood 77:2515-2523, 1991.
78. Truitt RL, Atasoylu AA: Contribution of CD4[+] and CD8[+] T cells to graft-vs-host disease and graft-vs-leukemia reactivity after transplantation of MHC-compatible bone marrow. Bone Marrow Transplant 8:51-58, 1991.
79. OKunewick JP, Kociban DL, Machen LL, et al: The role of CD4 and CD8 T-cells in the graft-vs-leukemia response in Rauscher murine leukemia. Bone Marrow Transplant 8:445-452, 1991.

80. Sykes M, Abraham VS, Harty MW, et al: IL-2 reduces graft-versus-host disease and preserves a graft-versus-leukemia effect by selectively inhibiting CD4$^+$ T cell activity. J Immunol 150:197-205, 1993.
81. Adler A, Chervenick PA, Whiteside TL, et al: Interleukin 2 induction of lymphokine-activated killer (LAK) activity in the peripheral blood and bone marrow of acute leukemia patients. I. Feasibility of LAK generation in adult patients with active disease and in remission. Blood 71:709-716, 1988.
82. Gottlieb DJ, Prentice HG, Heslop HE, et al: Effects of recombinant interleukin-2 administration on cytotoxic function following high-dose chemo-radiotherapy for hematological malignancy. Blood 74:2335-2342, 1989.
83. Delmon L, Ythier P, Moingeon P, et al: Characterization of antileukemia cells' cytotoxic effector function: Implications for monitoring natural killer responses following allogeneic bone marrow transplantation. Transplantation 42:252-256, 1986.
84. Heslop HE, Gottlieb DJ, Reittie JE, et al: Spontaneous and interleukin-2 induced secretion of tumor necrosis factor and gamma interferon following autologous marrow transplantation or chemotherapy. Br J Haematol 72:122-126, 1989.
85. Weiss L, Reich S, Slavin S: Use of recombinant human interleukin-2 in conjunction with bone marrow transplantation as a model for control of minimal residual disease in malignant hematological disorders. I. Treatment of murine leukemia in conjunction with allogeneic bone marrow transplantation and IL-2- activated cell-mediated immunotherapy. Cancer Invest 10:19-26, 1992.
86. Van Lochem E, de Gast B, Goulmy E: In vitro separation of host specific graft-versus-host and graft-versus-leukemia cytotoxic T cell activities. Bone Marrow Transplant 10:181-183, 1992.
87. Frassoni F, Sessarego M, Bacigalupo A, et al: Competition between recipient and donor cells after bone marrow transplantation for chronic myelogenous leukemia. Br J Haematol 69:471-475, 1988.
88. Collins RH, Rogers ZR, Bennet M, et al: Hematologic relapse of chronic myelogenous leukemia following allogeneic bone marrow transplantation: Apparent graft-versus-leukemia effect following abrupt discontinuation of immunosuppression. Bone Marrow Transplant 10:391-395, 1992.
89. Kolb JH, Mittermuller J, Clemm C, et al: Donor leukocyte transfusions for treatment of recurrent chronic myelogenous leukemia in marrow transplant patients. Blood 76:2462-2465, 1990.

90. Drobyski WR, Roth MS, Thibodeau SN, et al: Molecular remission occurring after donor leukocyte infusions for the treatment of relapsed chronic myelogenous leukemia after allogeneic bone marrow transplantation. Bone Marrow Transplant 10:301-304, 1992.

91. Jiang YZ, Kanfer EJ, Macdonald D, et al: Graft-versus-leukaemia following allogeneic bone marrow transplantation: Emergence of cytotoxic T lymphocytes reacting to host leukaemia cells. Bone Marrow Transplant 8:253-258, 1991.

92. DeVita VT Jr, Hellman S, Rosenberg SA: Biological Therapy of Cancer. Philadelphia, J.B. Lippincott, 1991.

93. Greenberg PD, Reusser P, Goodrich JM, et al: Development of a treatment regimen for human cytomegalovirus (CMV) infection in bone marrow transplantation recipients by adoptive transfer of donor-derived CMV-specific T cell clones expanded in vitro. Ann N Y Acad Sci 636:184-195, 1991.

94. Korngold R, Wettstein PJ: Immunodominance in the graft-vs-host disease T cell response to minor histocompatibility antigens. J Immunol 145:4079-4088, 1990.

95. Hauch M, Gazzola MV, Small T, et al: Anti-leukemia potential of interleukin-2 activated natural killer cells after bone marrow transplantation for chronic myelogenous leukemia. Blood 75:2250- 2262, 1990.

96. Niederwieser D, Gastl G, Rumpold H, et al: Rapid reappearance of large granular lymphocytes (LGL) with concurrent reconstitution of natural killer (NK) activity after human marrow transplantation. Br J Haematol 65:301-305, 1987.

97. Drobyski WR, Piaskowski V, Ash RC, et al: Preservation of lymphokine-activated killer activity following T cell depletion of human bone marrow. Transplantation 50:625-632, 1990.

98. Drobyski WR, McOlash L, Ash RC, et al: Comparative analysis of T-cell depletion techniques: Implications for the antileukemic efficacy of T-cell depleted allogeneic bone marrow transplantation. Blood 78(Suppl 1):227a, 1991. Abstract.

99. Apperley JF, Jones L, Hale G, et al: Bone marrow transplantation for patients with chronic myeloid leukaemia: T cell depletion with Campath-1 reduces the incidence of graft-versus-host disease but may increase the risk of leukaemia relapse. Bone Marrow Transplant 1:53-66, 1986.

100. Fisch P, Malkovsky M, Kovats S, et al: Recognition by human Vγ9/Vδ2 T cells of a GroEL homolog on Daudi Burkitt's lymphoma cells. Science 250:1269-1273, 1990.

101. Moretta L, Pende D, Bottino C, et al: Human CD3⁺4⁻8⁻WT31⁻ T lymphocyte populations expressing the putative T cell receptor

gamma gene product. A limiting dilution and clonal analysis. Eur J Immunol 17:1229-1234, 1987.

102. Ciccone E, Viale 0, Bottino C, et al: Antigen recognition by human T cell receptor gamma positive lymphocytes. Specific lysis of allogeneic cells after activation in mixed lymphocyte culture. J Exp Med 167:1517-1522, 1988.

103. Kabelitz D, Bender A, Schondelmair S, et al: A large fraction of human peripheral blood gamma/delta+ T cells is activated by *Mycobacterium tuberculosis* but not by its 65 kD heat shock protein. J Exp Med 171:667-679, 1990.

104. Kozbor D, Trinchieri G, Monos DA, et al: Human gamma/delta+ T lymphocytes recognize tetanus toxoid in an MHC-restricted fashion. J Exp Med 169:1847-1851, 1989.

105. Biassoni R, Ferrini S, Prigione I, et al: Activated CD3⁻ CD16⁺ natural killer cells express a subset of the lymphokine genes that are induced in activated TCR α/β⁺ and γ/δ⁺ T cells. Scand J Immunol 33:247-252, 1991.

106. Ferrini S, Bottino C, Biassoni R, et al.: Characterization of CD3⁺ CD4⁻ CD8⁻ clones expressing the putative T cell receptor gamma gene product. J Exp Med 166:277-282, 1987.

107. Viale M, Ferrini S, Bacigalupo A: TCR γ/δ positive lymphocytes after allogeneic bone marrow transplantation. Bone Marrow Transplant 10:249-253, 1992.

108. Urban JL, Schreiber H: Tumor Antigens. Annu Rev Immunol 10:617-644, 1992.

109. Collins SJ: *Bcr/abl* structure and expression in chronic myelogenous leukemia chronic phase and blast phase. In A Deisseroth and RB Arlinghaus (eds): Chronic Myelogenous Leukemia: Molecular Approaches to Research and Therapy. Volume 13. New York, NY, Marcel Dekker, 1991, p 253.

110. Peace DJ, Chen W, Nelson H, et al: T cell recognition of transforming proteins encoded by mutated ras proto-oncogenes. J Immunol 146:2059-2065, 1991.

111. Campbell MJ, Carroll W, Kon S, et al: Idiotype vaccination against murine B cell lymphoma: Humoral and cellular responses elicited by tumor-derived immunoglobulin M and its molecular subunits. J Immunol 139:2825-2833, 1987.

112. Greenberg PD, Klarnet J, Kern DE: Therapy of disseminated tumors by adoptive transfer of specifically immune T-cells. Prog Exp Tumor Res 32:104-127, 1988.

113. Greenberg PD: Adoptive T cell therapy of tumors: Mechanisms operative in the recognition and elimination of tumor cells. Adv Immunol 49:281-355, 1991.

114. Green WR: Recognition of G_{IX}-linked minor histocompatibility antigens by H-2-restricted cytotoxic T lymphocytes from C57BL/6-G_{IX}^+ mice: An approach to mapping the genes controlling G_{IX}. J Immunol 128:920-925, 1982.

115. Weiden PL, Horowitz MM: Graft-vs-leukemia effects in clinical bone marrow transplantation. In SJ Burakoff, HJ Deeg, J Ferrara, K Atkinson (eds): Graft-vs.-Host Disease: Immunology, Pathophysiology, and Treatment. New York, NY, Marcel Dekker, 1990, pp 691-708.

116. Krensky AM, Sanchez-Madrid F, Robbins E, et al: The functional significance, distribution, and structure of LFA-1, LFA-2, and LFA-3: Cell surface antigens associated with CTL-target interactions. J Immunol 131:611-616, 1983.

117. Figdor CG, van Kooyk Y, Keizer GD: On the mode of action of LFA-1. Immunol Today 11:277-280, 1990.

118. Trinchieri G, Perussia B: Human natural killer cells: Biologic and pathologic aspects. Lab Invest 50:489-513, 1984.

119. Imamura N, Kuramoto A: Natural killer activity is not dependent on the CD3-Ti T-cell receptor antigen complex. Blood 72:1837-1838, 1988. Letter.

120. Nitta T, Yagita H, Sato K, et al: Involvement of CD56 (NKH-1/Leu-19 antigen) as an adhesion molecule in natural killer-target cell interaction. J Exp Med 170:1757-1761, 1989.

121. Oblakowski P, Bello-Fernandez C, Reittie JE, et al: Possible mechanisms of selective killing of myeloid leukemic blast cells by lymphokine-activated killer cells. Blood 77:1996-2001, 1991.

122. Dustin ML, Springer TA: Lymphocyte function-associated antigen-1 (LFA-1) interaction with intercellular adhesion molecule-1 (ICAM-1) is one of at least three mechanisms for lymphocyte adhesion to cultured endothelial cells. J Cell Biol 107:321-331, 1988.

123. Schouten HC, Sizoo W, van't Veer MB, et al: Incomplete chimerism in erythroid, myeloid and B lymphocyte lineage after T cell-depleted allogeneic bone marrow transplantation. Bone Marrow Transplant 3:407-412, 1988.

124. Roy DC, Tantravahi R, Murray C, et al: Natural history of mixed chimerism after bone marrow transplantation with CD6-depleted allogeneic marrow: A stable equilibrium. Blood 75:296-304, 1990.

125. Lawler M, Humphries P, McCann SR: Evaluation of mixed chimerism by in vitro amplification of dinucleotide repeat sequences using the polymerase chain reaction. Blood 77:2504-2514, 1991.

126. Sprent J, Lo D, Gao EK, et al: T cell selection in the thymus. Immunol Rev 101:173-190, 1988.
127. Wilson DB: Idiotypic regulation of T cells in graft-versus- host disease and autoimmunity. Immunol Rev 107:159-177, 1989.
128. Sykes M, Eisenthal A, Sachs D: Mechanism of protection from graft-vs-host disease in murine mixed allogeneic chimeras. I. Development of a null cell population suppressive of cell-mediated lympholysis responses and derived from the syngeneic bone marrow component. J Immunol 140:2903-2911, 1988.
129. Qin SX, Cobbold S, Benjamin R, et al: Induction of classical transplantation tolerance in the adult. J Exp Med 169:779-794, 1989.
130. Truitt RL, Horowitz MM, Atasoylu AA, et al: Graft-versus-leukemia effect of allogeneic bone marrow transplantation: Clinical and experimental aspects of late leukemia relapse. In THM Stewart (ed): Cellular Immune Mechanisms and Tumor Dormancy. Boca Raton, Fla, CRC Press, 1992, pp 111-128.
131. Levite M, Reisner Y: Development of tolerance to donor type and host type H-2 antigens following transplantation of allogeneic bone marrow in mice. Bone Marrow Transplant 6:37-44, 1990.
132. Perreault C, Belanger R, Gyger M, et al: The mechanism of graft-host-tolerance in murine radiation chimeras transplanted across minor histocompatibility barriers. Bone Marrow Transplant 4:83-87, 1989.
133. Perreault C, Allard A, Brochu S, et al: Studies of immunologic tolerance to host minor histocompatibility antigens following allogeneic bone marrow transplantation in mice. Bone Marrow Transplant 6:127-135, 1990.
134. Sykes M, Bukhari Z, Sachs DH: Graft-versus-leukemia effect using mixed allogeneic bone marrow transplantation. Bone Marrow Transplant 4:465-474, 1989.
135. Sykes M, Romick ML, Sachs DH: Interleukin 2 prevents graft-vs-host disease without diminishing the graft-vs-leukemia effect of allogeneic lymphocytes. Proc Natl Acad Sci U S A 87:5633-5637, 1990.
136. Abraham VS, Sachs DH, Sykes M: The mechanism of protection from GVHD mortality by IL-2. III. Early reductions in donor T cell subsets and expansion of a $CD3^+ CD4^- CD8^-$ cell population. J Immunol 148:3746-3752, 1992.
137. Bortin MM, Truitt RL, Rimm AA, et al: Graft versus leukemia reactivity induced by alloimmunisation without augmentation of graft versus host reactivity. Nature 281:490-491, 1979.

138. Truitt RL, Shih CCY, Rimm AA, et al: Alloimmunization of H-2-compatible donors for adoptive immunotherapy of leukemia: Role of H-2, Mls and non-H-2 antigens. In A Fefer, AL Goldstein (eds): The Potential Role of T Cells in Cancer Therapy. New York, NY, Raven Press, 1982, pp 21-30.

139. Halle-Pannenko 0, Pritchard LL, Bruley-Rosset M: Abrogation of the lethal graft-vs-host reaction developed to non-H-2 antigens: Involvement of T suppressor cells distinct from veto cells. Eur J Immunol 17:1751-1755, 1987.

140. Bruley-Rosset M, Miconnet I, Canon C, et al: Mls^a generated suppressor cells. I. Suppression is mediated by double negative (CD3$^+$ CD5$^+$ CD4$^-$ CD8$^-$) $\alpha\beta$ T cell receptor bearing cells. J Immunol 145:4046-4052, 1990.

141. Pritchard LL, Huchet R, Bruley-Rosset M, et al: Induction and suppression of delayed-type hypersensitivity to non-MHC antigens during lethal graft-versus-host reaction. J Immunol 149:45-52, 1992.

142. Truitt RL, McCabe CM, Weiler MB and Johnson BJ: Contribution of CD4$^+$, CD8$^+$, and NKI.1$^+$ cells to antileukemia (GVL) and antihost (GVH) reactions after allogeneic bone marrow transplantation. J Cell Biochem Suppl 17D:118, 1993. Abstract #NZ 317.

Chapter 2

Immunomodulation in Autologous Bone Marrow Transplantation: Experimental Approaches

Bishan S. Charak, M.D., Udit N. Verma, M.D., Amitabha Mazumder, M.D.

Autologous bone marrow transplantation (BMT) permits the delivery of high doses of chemotherapy and/or radiotherapy to patients with cancer who either do not have a matched donor or are unfit for allogeneic BMT. This results in the cure of cancer in some patients whose disease is not responsive to conventional salvage therapies. However, autologous BMT is followed by a high relapse rate even in tumors that exhibit a linear response to chemo-radiotherapy. This has been explained on the basis of two broad issues inherently afflicting an autologous BMT situation:

1. presence of viable tufmor cells in the autograft even during the morphological remission of leukemias and some solid tumors; and
2. absence of an immune response against host tumor unlike that seen following allogeneic BMT.

From: Spitzer T, Mazumder A: Immunotherapy and Bone Marrow Transplantation. Armonk, NY, Futura Publishing Co., Inc., © 1995.

Strategies aimed at eradication of tumor cells from the autograft resulted in the development of several purging techniques. In vitro purging of the bone marrow (BM) by physical (magnetic beads), pharmacological (chemotherapeutic agents) and immunological (monoclonal antibodies) means is widely practiced. All these approaches, when employed alone or in combination, result in significant eradication of tumor cells from the BM. However, the influence of in vitro purging of BM on the disease outcome has not been clear. Although presence of tumor cells in the BM is an important cause of a relapse, relapses take place even when purged BM is used for autologous BMT. This suggests that relapses following autologous BMT are related, in part, to the residual disease in the body of the patient escaping the high dose chemo-radiotherapy.

Hypotheses about reactivation of residual disease have prompted workers to develop approaches to stimulate the host immune system. It has been hoped that the host immune system could serve as a surveillance mechanism that would check the proliferation of minimal disease, and thus prevent a relapse. These approaches have resulted in the development of strategies designed to induce what has been termed as a graft-versus-tumor (GVT) effect.

Several immunomodulators have been employed with the aim of induction of a GVT effect following autologous BMT. These have included interleukin (IL)-2, interferon (IFN), cyclosporine A (CsA), granulocyte macrophage-colony stimulating factor (GM-CSF), monoclonal antibodies (MAB) and tumor vaccines. IL-2 and IFN have been known to induce cytotoxic cells with major histocompatibility complex (MHC)-unrestricted cytotoxicity. IL-2 results in the proliferation of T cells and natural killer (NK) cells, and also induces the secretion of secondary cytokines such as IFN and tumor necrosis factor (TNF). All of these processes result in potent antitumor effect. IFN stimulates NK-cell function, enhances the expression of MHC-antigens on tumor cells and promotes the antitumor activities of macrophages. CsA has been reported to interfere with the T-cell differentiation in the thymus resulting in the release of autoreactive cells in the peripheral circulation; these cells have also been shown to possess an antitumor effect. GM-CSF has been reported to induce antibody dependent cellular cytotoxicity (ADCC) via stimulation of granulocytes, lymphocytes and monocytes. MAB achieve a high concentration at the tumor sites following irradiation. When used with IL-2 or GM-CSF, they induce a potent GVT effect via ADCC. Tumor cell vaccines are being developed to ensure a long term immunity to the tumor. The following sections describe some of the data regarding the induction of GVT effect in preclinical, syngeneic BMT models.

Interleukin-2

Murine Studies

IL-2 is a T-cell growth factor; it leads to proliferation of these cells both in vitro and in vivo.[1,2] Incubation of lymphocytes with IL-2 results in the generation of a population of cells known as lymphokine-activated killer (LAK) cells.[3] LAK cells show antitumor activity against a wide variety of tumors in an MHC- unrestricted manner.[4,5] LAK cells can be generated from all lymphoid tissues, viz., peripheral blood, BM, thymus, spleen, lymph nodes and thoracic duct.[6,7] LAK cells has been shown to have a purging effect on the tumor cells contaminating the BM.[8] However, the ability of IL-2 to generate killer cells within the BM could eliminate the need for generation of LAK cells on a large scale and be of potentially greater value; it could eradicate the minimal residual disease in the autograft, while still retaining the function of reconstitution of the hematopoietic system. In addition, the killer cells could eradicate the residual disease in the host, as the tumor burden is minimal following preparative therapy for autologous BMT.

Generation of Killer Cells in the Bone Marrow

Incubation of murine BM with IL-2 in vitro results in the generation of killer cells with potent cytotoxicity against NK-sensitive as well as NK-resistant tumor cells.[7] The cytotoxic potential of IL-2-activated bone marrow (ABM) increases with the duration of incubation with IL-2, peaks around the fourth or fifth day, and then starts declining slowly. On a per cell basis, the cytotoxicity of ABM cells is superior to that of spleen LAK cells both in vitro and in vivo.[7,9] Interestingly, under similar conditions of in vitro culture, the cytotoxic potential of ABM cells declines much more slowly than that of LAK cells. Finally, the IL-2 requirements of ABM cells to maintain antitumor effect in vivo was at least 10 times less than that of LAK cells.[9] Thus, low dose IL-2 therapy following BMT with ABM could induce a significant GVT effect. Since the toxicity of IL-2 therapy is related to its dose, this approach could help minimize the IL-2-induced toxicity. Recently, Charak et al. have shown that ABM can be generated from BM that has leukemic contamination; this ABM showed antileukemic effect both in vitro and in vivo.[10] However, the ability of IL-2 to generate killer cells from leukemic BM was inversely related to the degree of leukemic infiltration. This observation suggests that IL-2-activation of BM from patients with leukemia in remission (when the leukemic infiltration is minimal) might be able to eradicate the contaminating leukemia and serve as a purging strategy.

The exact phenotype of the ABM cells is not known at present. It has been reported that the precursors of ABM cells are double negative cluster designation (CD3+, CD4-, CD8-),[11,12] while some of the effectors acquire the Thy-1 marker.[7] Interestingly, some ABM clones display T-cell receptors, are positive for CD3 and NK markers, are negative for CD4 and CD8 markers and have a high affinity IL-2 receptor on the same cells. Besides, the depletion of NK cells from the ABM that has been generated over a short period of time (1 to 3 days) does not result in a significant loss of cytotoxicity. All of these characteristics suggest that the ABM cells may be different from conventional LAK cells.

Effect on Hematopoiesis

IL-2 therapy has been reported to cause hematologic changes including anemia and thrombocytopenia in cancer patients.[13] Others have reported an increase in the circulating hematopoietic precursors following IL-2 therapy.[14,15] Based on the in vitro studies, conflicting data have been published regarding the effect of IL-2 and LAK cells on BM progenitor cell activity (PCA). Some reports suggest that IL-2 and LAK cells inhibit,[16-19] while others suggest that they spare the PCA of BM in vitro.[20-22] Although ABM contains potent cytotoxic cells against tumors, failure of engraftment following BMT with ABM could offset the benefits of the antitumor effect. However, most of the published data regarding the effect of IL-2 on the PCA of BM have been generated in vitro, and in vitro PCA does not predict the engraftment potential of BM.[23] Charak et al. have examined the effect of IL-2 and ABM on establishing hematopoiesis in a BMT setting.[24] In vitro incubation of BM for 1 to 3 days resulted in a progressive decline in its PCA; this was related to the duration of in vitro culture, and not to the presence or absence of IL-2 in the culture medium. The trafficking pattern of the ABM that was generated over 24 hours was comparable to that of the fresh BM. However, when BM was kept in culture for 2 or 3 days before being used for BMT, it remained trapped in extrahematopoietic sites (liver and lungs) for a long time, delaying its homing to hematopoietic sites.[24] This was probably related to alteration in the homing receptors on the BM cells. Generation of ABM over 24 hours results in significant cytotoxicity in vitro and in vivo.[7,9] Therefore, Mazumder's group have been employing ABM generated over 24 hours for their in vivo studies. BMT with such an ABM results in normal hematopoiesis both in a leukemic and a nonleukemic setting.[24,25] In addition, treatment with IL-2 immediately after BMT with ABM or with fresh bone marrow (FBM) did not interfere with reconstitution of the hematopoietic system. Regeneration of peripheral blood counts, BM cellularity and the PCA of the engrafted BM were comparable whether BMT was performed with FBM or ABM and whether or not IL-2 was administered after BMT.[24-26]

Induction of Graft-Versus-Tumor Effect

High dose IL-2 and infusion of large numbers of LAK cells have been reported to cause tumor regression,[27,28] but complete eradication of the tumor by these means is rare. Besides, high dose IL-2 therapy is associated with serious toxicity that offsets the improved survival achieved by greater tumor eradication.[28] It appears that the efficacy of immunotherapy is limited to the eradication of small tumor burden. From that perspective, autologous BMT provides an attractive setting for application of immunotherapy, as the residual disease escaping the preparative therapy in transplantation is minimum in the early posttransplant period. In addition, tumor cells exposed to chemotherapy have been reported to show increased susceptibility to lysis by immune defense cells.[29]

The role of IL-2 in inducing a GVT effect following syngeneic BMT for several solid tumors and leukemias has been examined. To a certain extent, the results vary for different tumor models and the experimental designs. Ackerstein et al. have shown that administration of IL-2 3 weeks after BMT with FBM resulted in greater GVT effect than IL-2 therapy instituted immediately after BMT.[30] This was explained on the basis of high antitumor effect of lymphocytes regenerating during the third week following BMT. This group employed a schedule of high dose (10^5 units three times a day for 5 days) IL-2 therapy.

Mazumder's group have examined extensively the role of IL-2 in the induction of a GVT effect against a wide variety of tumors.[7,9,10,25,31-33] Institution of IL-2 after BMT with FBM did not induce any GVT effect against solid tumors (a melanoma and a sarcoma),[7,9] or against acute myeloid leukemia (AML).[25,31,32] The GVT effect following BMT with ABM without IL-2 therapy was not different from the GVT effect of BMT with FBM, with or without IL-2 therapy. However, BMT with ABM followed immediately by IL-2 therapy for 7 days resulted in a potent GVT effect. This approach led to a significant control of dissemination of NK-resistant solid tumors,[7,9] and led to cure in a significant population of mice with AML.[25,31] Institution of IL-2 therapy even 1 to 3 weeks after BMT with FBM did not induce any GVT effect. On the other hand, when IL-2 therapy was delayed for 1 to 3 weeks after BMT with ABM, there was a progressive decline in the cure rate, suggesting a loss of GVT effect.[31] When institution of IL-2 was delayed after BMT with ABM, many animals died because of relapse of AML even before completion of therapy.

The exact mechanisms of induction and maintenance of GVT effect in this system are yet to be defined. However, these studies have brought up several important issues. IL-2 by itself was incapable of generating cells with antileukemic effect in vivo. IL-2 has been used at variable intervals following autologous BMT.[34,35] It increases the NK activity and in an occasional case, spontaneous LAK activity. These data have been considered to represent an antitumor response, and this approach has been expected to reduce the relapse rate following autologous BMT. A recent study has shown that increase in the NK activity is a function of duration of IL-2 therapy and can be generated by institution of IL-2 therapy any time after BMT with FBM.[10] However, IL-2-induced NK activity did not translate into increased GVT effect in vivo.[36] Generation of endogenous LAK cells requires the administration of very high doses of IL-2 that are often toxic.[28] On the other hand, the schedule of IL-2 therapy (10^4 units twice daily for 7 days) employed in our studies was absolutely nontoxic.[24] Administrations of low dose IL-2 following BMT with ABM, however, seems to maintain the antitumor effect of these killer cells in vivo.

Another important aspect of these studies was that in the absence of IL-2 therapy, ABM cells did not induce any GVT effect.[25,31] It appears that like LAK cells, ABM cells are highly dependent on a constant supply of IL-2 for their cytotoxic function in vivo. In the absence of exogenous IL-2, they lose their cytotoxic potential and behave like inactivated BM cells. This was possibly the reason for loss of GVT effect when IL-2 therapy was delayed following BMT with ABM. Thus, for optimum GVT effect, the ABM and IL-2 act as complements to each other. Maximum tolerated doses of IL-2 result in serum concentrations (5 to 10 U/mL)[37] that are far below those required for generation of ABM in vitro.[7] Therefore, it seems necessary to prime the BM with IL-2 in vitro before autologous BMT. Low levels of IL-2 achieved by parenteral IL-2 therapy instituted immediately following autologous BMT may be enough to maintain an antitumor effect that could eradicate the residual disease.

These studies also showed that IL-2 therapy immediately after BMT was safe. The maximum tolerated dose of IL-2 in a BMT setting was at least 10 times more than that in a non-BMT setting.[10] The exact reason for this difference is not known. IL-2-induced toxicity has been related to the proliferation of lymphocytes resulting in encroachment on contiguous tissues, direct lysis of tissues by LAK cells and effect of the secondary cytokines induced by IL-2.[38-40] A recent study has shown that IL-2-induced toxicity is related to activated NK cells, while the antitumor effect is related to Lyt-2+, L3T4+ cells.[40] Our studies have shown that depletion of NK cells from ABM generated over 1 day does not result in loss of antitumor effect in vitro. These observations suggest that BMT with ABM and IL-2 therapy retains the antitumor effect but is not afflicted by the toxicity related to conventional LAK cells/IL-2 therapy.

BMT with ABM and/or IL-2 therapy did not cause graft-versus-host disease (GVHD).[25,26,31] This may be partly because of low numbers of T cells in the murine BM and partly because it was a syngeneic system. Moreover, IL-2 has actually been reported to generate cells capable of overriding the GVHD.[41,42]

The GVT effect generated by IL-2 therapy even after BMT with ABM, does not confer long-term immunity to the tumor. When cured, leukemic mice were rechallenged with leukemia in the late posttransplant period; their survival was not different from those mice that had not undergone a previous exposure to leukemia and BMT with ABM.[31] Further studies need to be carried out to generate killer cells that can maintain a function of long-term surveillance.

The exact mechanisms of enhanced GVT effect following BMT with ABM and IL-2 are not known at present. Improved GVT may be related to eradication of residual disease by cellular mechanisms.[10] IL-2 therapy after autologous BMT has been reported to induce the secretion of IFN and TNF[43] Both of these cytokines have direct antitumor effect, as well as synergize with IL-2 in the generation of killer cells from the BM.[44] IL-2 therapy has also been reported to induce ADCC.[33,45] Application of MAB therapy in an autologous BMT setting could be of potentially great value, as irradiation has been reported to enhance the MAB uptake by tumor tissue.[46] A better understanding of the biological processes working in concert with IL-2 will help develop strategies with more potent antitumor effect. This may also result in a better reconstitution of the immune system that might prevent delayed relapses following autologous BMT.

Human Studies

IL-2 has been widely used both in BMT, as well as in nontransplant situations. However, very few studies have evaluated its influence on the generation of killer cells from the BM with the aim of using the same BM for autologous BMT. Ability to generate significant killer cell activity in the BM without loss of its engraftment potential would constitute an important strategy in employing biotherapy in clinical autologous BMT.

Generation of Killer Cells in the Bone Marrow

Like murine BM, in vitro incubation of human BM with IL-2 leads to the generation of killer cells with potent antitumor effect in vitro.[22,24,47,48] The cytotoxic potential of ABM generated from patients with active disease is lower than the cytotoxicity of ABM generated from BM in remission.[47] In contrast to peripheral blood LAK cells, which take 5 to 7 days for generation of significant cytotoxicity, ABM can be generated over a short period of time (eg, 1 day).[22] This is of particular importance in autologous BMT, as a brief in vitro incubation will not lead to a significant loss of progenitor cells. The ABM cells show potent cytotoxicity against a variety of tumor cell lines and fresh tumor cells in an MHC-unrestricted manner.[22,47] Under similar culture conditions, the in vitro cytotoxic potential of ABM cells is greater than that of peripheral blood LAK cells on a per cell basis.[22,49] The requirement of IL-2 for generation of ABM cells is much lower than for LAK cells. Also, if deprived of IL-2 in vitro, the ABM cells maintain their cytotoxicity for a longer period than LAK cells.

The exact phenotype and mechanisms of lysis by the ABM cells have not been defined so far. Preliminary studies in our laboratory suggest that the precursor and effector of ABM is a T cell. Depletion of NK cells from ABM generated over 24 hours did not result in a significant loss of cytotoxicity. A recent study has shown that treatment of BM with CAMPATH-1, a MAB against T cells results in a significant depletion of ABM precursors.[50] This indicates that IL-2 therapy after BMT with T-cell-depleted BM may not be able to induce a GVT effect.

Generation of killer cells within the BM could prove to be of great benefit in the elimination of residual disease. It provides a tool for purging the autograft in vitro. The killer cells infused to the patient could also eradicate the residual tumor in the patient's body. To this end, it has been shown that IL-2 does not promote the growth of human leukemic cells.[51] IL-2 activation of BM for 1 or 3 days results in a significant purging of the contaminating leukemic cells in the BM.[22] Since longer incubation of BM in vitro results in greater loss of BM cells, IL-2 activation of BM should be preferably carried out for 1 day for clinical application of ABM. Many other cytokines have been known to influence the ability of IL-2 in generating killer cells from the BM and thus, its purging potential.[44] IL-1, IFN and TNF synergize with IL-2 and eradicate a much higher contamination of leukemia from the BM than is possible with IL-2 alone.[44,48] However, several other issues need to be addressed before formulating a purging protocol involving multiple cytokines. TNF and IFN have both been reported to suppress hematopoiesis.[52,53] IL-1 receptors have been demonstrated on the surface of myeloid leukemic cells from some patients.[54] Thus, further studies must be performed to develop a purging protocol involving a cytokine other than IL-2.

Interleukin-2 Activation of Bone Marrow in Long-Term Culture

The marrows of patients with chronic myeloid leukemia (CML), placed into Dexter type long-term bone marrow culture (LTC), over time produce increasing numbers of Philadelphia chromosome negative (Ph[1-]) hematopoietic cells.[55,56] The culture environment could provide growth advantage to Ph[1-] hematopoietic precursors.[57] LTC could be a better strategy for IL-2 activation of the marrow, as it can provide sufficient time for generation of full cytotoxic potential of the marrow[58] This can lead to more complete in vitro purging and potent graft-versus-leukemia (GVL) effect once it is transplanted back to the patients. However, culture conditions need to be optimized in such a way so as to maintain the reconstituting ability of cultured marrow.

BM from normal donors placed in LTC in the presence of IL-2 (1000 U/mL) develops marked cytotoxicity against a variety of tumor cell targets.[59] This cytotoxicity, as tested against A375 (melanoma), K562 (CML), Daudi (Burkitt) cell lines, was maintained up to 3 weeks. The inhibitory influence of hydrocortisone present in LTC medium was evident only at day 7. Thereafter, the cytotoxicity generated in cells cultured with or without hydrocortisone was comparable.

Hematopoietic precursor cell numbers were evaluated by enumerating day 14 colonies in methylcellulose cultures. No decline in number of clonogenic cells was seen in 7-day-old IL-2 cultures, as compared to non-IL-2 cultures or FBM. However, after 2 weeks a rapid decline in the number of clonogenic cells was seen in IL-2 cultures.

Based on the above findings and the feasibility of a clinically applicable protocol, the in vitro purging ability of IL-2 cultures was tested in 10-day-old cultures. Complete eradication of A375 and CEM (T cell acute lymphoblastic leukemia [T-ALL]) cells was seen after a 10-day culture of marrow contaminated with these cell lines at BM to tumor cell ratios of 100:1 or 10:1. No residual clonable K562 cells were seen after a 10-day IL-2 culture of marrow contaminated with these cells at BM to tumor cell ratio of 100:1. However, at higher contaminating ratio (10:1), complete eradication was seen only with 2 out of the 5 marrows tested; in the remaining 3, a marked decrease was seen in number of clonogenic K562 cells.[59]

Encouraged by these results, the purging efficacy of IL-2- stimulated LTC was tested with CML marrow. BMs from 4 Ph[1+] CML patients were placed in LTC with or without IL-2. After a 10-day culture, no Ph[1+] metaphases were detectable in the BM cultures with IL-2, as compared to control LTCs in which the majority of metaphases were still positive for Ph[1].

Further experiments were done in the murine model to test antitumor activity and reconstituting ability of IL-2-stimulated LTC (U.N. Verma, A. Mazumder, unpublished data). C1498-induced leukemic marrow from C57Bl/6 mice was harvested at different intervals after induction of leukemia to represent variable leukemic load in the marrow. This leukemic marrow was given back to normal syngeneic mice after 10 days of culture with or without IL-2. Mice receiving BM with minimal leukemia and cultured with IL-2 for 10 days did not develop leukemia; in contrast, 100% mortality was seen in the group receiving control marrow. However, at heavy leukemic loads, this survival advantage was lost. These results indicate that at low leukemic loads there was complete eradication of leukemic cells.

To test the reconstituting ability of IL-2 cultured marrow, lethally irradiated C57Bl/6 mice were given back IL-2 or control cultured syngeneic marrow. Both groups of mice given back 10 day cultured marrow with or without IL-2 were rescued.

These studies indicate that 10 days culture of BM in the presence of IL-2 under Dexter type culture conditions leads to generation of potent antitumor cytotoxicity without loss of engraftment potential. In the setting of autologous BMT, this technique could be used for generation of antitumor effectors which can mediate in vitro purging and in vivo GVL effect.

Effect on Hematopoiesis

Initial studies suggested that IL-2 and LAK cells inhibit the PCA of BM in vitro.[16-19] However, subsequent studies have failed to substantiate these findings.[20,21] Charak et al. have shown that IL-2-activation of BM does not impair its PCA.[22,44] In vitro PCA is a poor predictor of engraftment.[23] Nevertheless, we have shown that BMT with IL-2-activated fresh or frozen BM results in normal hematopoiesis both in leukemic as well as nonleukemic settings in mice.[10,25,31] The ABM has recently been used in a patient with AML; it led to normal hematopoiesis.[60] So far, three patients with refractory lymphomas who had received extensive chemotherapy and irradiation for their disease have undergone autologous BMT with ABM at our center. All of them engrafted within 4 weeks.

If ABM undergoes the procedures of freezing and thawing, it loses its cytotoxic activity.[22,31] Therefore, for clinical application, ABM has to be generated after thawing the BM prior to infusion. The frozen BM cells are fragile, undergo lysis after thawing, and release lysosomal enzymes which cause clumping and cell loss.[61] Besides, generation of ABM for clinical use would require the handling of large amounts of culture medium. Charak et al. have recently described a technique for handling the frozen BM on a large scale.[62] Addition of DNAse to the BM concentrate before freezing or immediately after thawing, and addition of heparin (and IL-2) in a serum-free medium completely abolished the clump formation, resulting in a significant cytotoxicity and no loss of PCA.[62] This technique ensured the recovery of 78% of the mononuclear cells after complete processing following 24-hour activation of the autograft with IL-2. This method could be of potential benefit in immunomodulation of a frozen stock of BM after thawing, even with agents other than IL-2.

Cyclosporine A in Autologous Bone Marrow Transplantation

CsA is a potent immunosuppressive agent widely used following solid organ transplantation and allogeneic BMT. Paradoxically, when used in a syngeneic BMT setting in Lewis rats, CsA leads to the development of GVHD.[63,64] CsA therapy causes immunopathological changes in the thymus, including medullary involution, loss of Hassal's corpuscles, and decreased expression of Ia antigen.[65] These changes are irreversible if the thymus has been irradiated and thus, interfere with the intrathymic differentiation of T cells.[63,64,66] Furthermore, CsA has been reported to inhibit apoptosis within the thymus, resulting in the release of highly autoreactive lymphocytes into the peripheral circulation.[67,68] However, the exact mechanisms of CsA-induced GVHD remain to be defined.[69] The issues of induction, mechanism and possible role of syngeneic GVHD in preventing tumor relapse are discussed in greater detail in chapter 3.

Interestingly, the autoreactive cells, which are generated by CsA therapy following autologous BMT, have also been shown to have antitumor effect in vitro.[70] Unfortunately, the cytotoxic potential of these cells is related to the expression of Ia antigen on the tumor cell surface. They do not show any cytotoxicity against tumors that do not express Ia antigen, thus limiting the wider applicability of this system. In addition, CsA therapy induces GVHD in a few, not all, strains of rats and mice.[71,72] Thus, this system is highly dependent on the immunological makeup of the host.

Mazumder's group have examined the role of a combination therapy with CsA and IL-2 against non-Ia-bearing tumors in a syngeneic BMT setting, in a strain of mice that do not develop GVHD following CsA therapy.[73] The rationale for combining these two agents was based on the data that CsA-generated T cells are highly responsive to IL-2 in vitro,[74] and IL-2 generates cells with MHC-unrestricted cytotoxicity from cells with similar phenotype as those generated after CsA. Thus, this system could be of potentially greater applicability than CsA alone. Besides, IL-2 therapy alone after BMT with FBM did not induce any GVT effect in our previous studies.[9,25,31]

Our data show that IL-2 or CsA alone, after BMT, did not induce increased antitumor effect, as compared to BMT alone, against a melanoma (B16) or an AML (C1498) in mice.[73] However, a combination of IL-2 and CsA after BMT significantly improved the antitumor effect, as compared to BMT alone. The combination therapy controlled the dissemination of both tumors, prolonged the survival of the mice, and improved the cure rate, as compared to BMT alone. The spleen cells harvested from mice undergoing IL-2 plus CsA therapy after BMT showed antitumor effect not only against the syngeneic tumor cells (B16 or C1498, both H-2^b tumors), but also against an allogeneic target (P815 mastocytoma, an H-2^d tumor) in vitro. This cytotoxicity could not be blocked by an Ia antibody and was not enhanced by increased expression of Ia antigen on the tumor cells.[73]

More interestingly, the antitumor effect generated in the primary tumor bearers could be adoptively transferred into secondary tumor bearers. Spleen cells harvested from mice undergoing IL-2 plus CsA therapy after BMT were infused into secondary tumor bearers; they led to a significant control of the tumors in the secondary recipients even in the absence of further IL-2 or CsA therapy. This effect was more pronounced in the secondary recipients that underwent chemo-radiotherapy. The exact reason for this phenomenon is not known. It is possible that chemo-radiotherapy abolished a host-suppressor mechanism, interrupted the tolerance to the tumor, and allowed the adoptively transferred effectors to manifest greater antitumor effect.[75-77] The final effector mechanisms operative in this system are not known. Preliminary data showed that the cellular components inhibiting the antitumor effect were comprised of asialo GM1[+] and Thy-1[+] cells.

Combination therapy with IL-2 and CsA following BMT in tumor-bearing mice did not induce GVHD.[67] This may be partly because the mouse strain (C57BL/6) used in that study is not prone to GVHD following CsA therapy,[71,72] and partly because IL-2 is known to stimulate cells capable of suppressing GVHD.[41,42] Conventionally, GVHD and GVT have been considered inseparable.[78] However, our study shows that different mechanisms may be operative in the development of these two processes and it may be possible to induce GVT without GVHD.[73]

Granulocyte Macrophage-Colony Stimulating Factor-Induced Antibody Dependent Cellular Cytotoxicity in Autologous Bone Marrow Transplantation

GM-CSF has been widely used following autologous BMT with the aim of hastening the myeloid recovery.[79,80] GM-CSF stimulates the proliferation of myeloid progenitors at different stages of differentiation, reduces the duration of severe neutropenia, and improves the function of mature neutrophils.[81-83] Thus, GM-CSF therapy reduces morbidity and mortality from infections related to severe neutropenia.

GM-CSF has also been reported to induce antitumor effect by stimulation of neutrophils, lymphocytes and monocytes.[84-86] The increase in the cytotoxic potential of monocytes has been reported to be due to the direct effect of GM-CSF, as well as via ADCC.[86,87] Since monocytes play an important role in defense against cancer, it is tempting to stimulate the monocytes for induction of GVT in autologous BMT.

Another attractive mode of therapy in autologous BMT is the treatment with MAB. Conventional treatment with MAB in patients with cancer has met with limited success due to failure of the antibody to achieve optimum concentration at the tumor sites and variable expression of tumor antigens on the cell surface.[88] Recent studies have shown that prior irradiation of the tumor significantly enhances the MAB uptake by the tumor tissue.[46] Thus, high concentrations of the MAB could be achieved on the residual disease in an autologous BMT setting.

Mazumder's group have recently examined the role of GM-CSF in inducing ADCC via BM macrophages.[89,90] They further evaluated the applicability of this approach in inducing a GVT effect in an autologous BMT setting. GM-CSF-induced ADCC in BM macrophages was evaluated against a murine melanoma (B16), a human melanoma (A375) and a human lymphoma (Raji) by employing tumor specific MAB.[90]

GM-CSF induced a potent ADCC against B16 melanoma both in vitro and in vivo.[89] Melanoma is a radioresistant tumor; BMT alone did not control its dissemination in mice. However, infusion of GM-CSF-activated BM macrophages in a BMT setting resulted in a marked reduction in the spread of tumors as well as prolonged the survival of the tumor-bearing mice.[89] Adoptive transfer of BM macrophages harvested from mice undergoing GM-CSF therapy resulted in a significant control of dissemination of tumor in the secondary recipients.[90] Once again, this effect was more manifest when the secondary recipients had received prior irradiation. These observations suggest that chemo-radiotherapy, employed as a preparative therapy for BMT, might have damaged a suppressor system, thus facilitating the efficacy of effector cells.[75-77]

Human GM-CSF induced a potent ADCC in the human BM macrophages against both of the tumors tested in vitro.[90] It also induced an antitumor effect against Raji tumor cells implanted in nude mice. Once again, the antitumor effect of GM-CSF-activated

BM macrophages was greater if the mice were injected with cyclophosphamide (CY) prior to infusion of macrophages.[90] Immunocytochemical studies confirmed increased localization of the antibody at the tumor site in mice exposed to CY. Our data showed that the GM-CSF-induced ADCC was specific in vitro. In addition, it could not be blocked by antibodies to TNF, IL-1, and MHC-I and -II antigens.[90] These data point to a great potential of GM-CSF in inducing a GVT in autologous BMT.

Future Directions

It is too early to derive inferences about the impact of IL-2 therapy used in clinical autologous BMT. Analyses of data from preclinical and clinical studies carried out by employing IL-2 therapy in resistant cancers in nontransplant situations have yielded encouraging information. However, although most tumors are sensitive to IL-2/LAK cell therapy both in vitro and in vivo, complete cures following this form of therapy have been rare. This may be related to the presence of large tumor burdens, low concentrations of IL-2 at every tumor site, inappropriate trafficking of killer cells to the tumor sites, suboptimal protocols employed, immunocompromised status of the host, or endogenous inhibitory influences. Autologous BMT provides an interesting situation as the residual disease is at its minimum and high dose chemo-radiotherapy might have rendered it susceptible to killer cells. Future studies should focus on enhancing the delivery of the IL-2 killer cell system to the tumor sites. This may be particularly possible by employing tumor-specific antibodies and exploiting the IL-2-induced ADCC. A recent study has shown that formation of an immunoconjugate of a MAB and IL-2 achieved high concentration at the tumor sites, while its concentration in normal tissues including blood, muscles, and heart, was much lower.[91] Such approaches need to be evaluated in autologous BMT.

Identification and purification of the effector cell population operative in the IL-2-generated killer cell system would be of immense benefit. While it will allow the delivery of specific killer cells, it may also shed some light on the inhibitory influences, especially in an in vivo situation. In addition, several other cytokines are known to influence the ability of IL-2 to generate killer cells. Use of an optimum combination of cytokines may help both by generating more potent antitumor cells, as well as by antagonizing the inhibitory influences.

The efficacy of IL-2 in vivo has been limited, in part, by its toxicity. New approaches need to be developed to overcome this problem. This will probably require slow delivery systems to maintain constant but low levels, combination with other cytokines, and use of cell populations with antitumor effect but limited toxicity. To this effect, IL-1 has been shown to reduce the IL-2 induced pulmonary toxicity.[92] Similarly, activated NK cells have been associated with toxicity, while L3+T4+ cells have been associated with IL-2-induced antitumor effect.[40] These systems need to be further defined for applicability in an autologous BMT setting.

The CsA-induced autoimmune syndrome has been associated with expression of MHC-antigens and limited antitumor effect. Preliminary preclinical data suggest that this system can be exploited to generate MHC-unrestricted antitumor effect both in transplant and nontransplant situations.[73,77] Future work should be carried out to define the cellular and humoral factors involved in this phenomenon. An understanding of the role of CsA in breaking the tolerance to self will clarify some of the mechanisms operative in this system.

Further work needs also to be carried out in optimizing and in detailed definition of GM-CSF-induced ADCC. Preliminary work shows that cellular interactions involving more than one type of cell population are operative in generating GM-CSF-induced ADCC. In addition, availability of MAB with wider spectrum of applicability in a clinical situation could offer great promise in this approach.

Most of the approaches currently being evaluated in the preclinical and clinical situations appear to be incapable of inducing a long term immunity to the tumor. Future studies need to develop tumor cell vaccines that could induce immune response against the residual tumor at the earliest, cause its rejection and thus, prevent a relapse. Future work will also see the application, in autologous BMT, of certain genes that could secrete antitumor factors and eradicate the residual disease.

In conclusion, immunomodulation in autologous BMT provides a uniquely attractive setting for improving the host immune defenses in general and inducing a GVT effect in particular. Preclinical studies have provided some insight into the mechanisms that can be possibly explored. Future work should focus on better understanding and optimization of these phenomena. Application of these approaches could then be translated into benefits in clinical situations.

References

1. Morgan DA, Ruscetti FW, Gallo R: Selective in vitro growth of T-lymphocytes from normal bone marrow. Science 193:1007-1008, 1976.
2. Ettinghausen SE, Lipford EH III, Mule JJ, et al: Systemic administration of recombinant interleukin-2 stimulates in vivo lymphoid cell proliferation in tissues. J Immunol 135:1488-1497, 1985.
3. Rosenstein M, Yron I, Kaufmann Y, et al: Lymphokine-activated killer cells: Lysis of fresh syngeneic natural killer resistant murine tumor cells by lymphocytes cultured in interleukin-2. Cancer Res 44:1946-1953, 1984.
4. Grimm EA, Rosenberg SA: The lymphokine activated killer cell phenomenon. Lymphokines 9:279-285, 1984.

5. Rosenberg SA: Lymphokine activated killer cells: A new approach to immunotherapy of cancer. J Natl Cancer Inst 75:595-603, 1985.

6. Grimm EA, Ramsey KM, Mazumder A, et al: Lymphokine-activated killer cell phenomenon-II precursor phenotype is serologically distinct from peripheral T lymphocytes, memory cytotoxic thymus-derived lymphocytes, and natural killer cells. J Exp Med 157: 884-897, 1983.

7. Agah R, Malloy B, Kerner M, et al: Generation and characterization of IL-2-activated bone marrow cells as a potent graft vs tumor effector in transplantation. J Immunol 143:3093- 3099, 1989.

8. Long GS, Hiserodt JC, Harnaha JB, et al: Lymphokine-activated killer cell purging of leukemia cells from bone marrow prior to syngeneic transplantation. Transplantation 46 :433-438, 1988.

9. Agah R, Malloy B, Kerner M, et al: Potent graft antitumor effect in natural killer-resistant disseminated tumors by transplantation of interleukin-2-activated syngeneic bone marrow in mice. Cancer Res 49:5959-5963, 1989.

10. Charak BS, Brynes RK, Chogyoji M, et al: Graft versus leukemia effect of interleukin-2-activated bone marrow: Correlation with eradication of residual disease. Transplantation 56:31-37, 1993.

11. Sykes M: Unusual T-cell population in adult murine bone marrow. Prevalence of CD3+ CD4- CD8- and αβ-TCR+ NK 1.1+ cells. J Immunol 146:3209-3215, 1990.

12. Sykes M, Hoyles KA, Romick ML, et al: In vitro and in vivo analysis of bone marrow-derived CD3+, CD4-, CD8-, NK 1.1+ cell lines. Cell Immunol 129:478-493, 1990.

13. Ettinghausen SE, Moore JG, White DE, et al: Hematologic effects of immunotherapy with lymphokine-activated killer cells and recombinant interleukin-2 in cancer patients. Blood 69: 1654-1660, 1987.

14. Schaafsma MR, Fibbe WE, van der Harst D, et al: Increased numbers of circulating hematopoietic progenitor cells after treatment with high-dose interleukin-2 in cancer patients. Br J Haematol 76:180-185, 1990.

15. Lafreniere R, Houwen B, Rankin C, et al: In vivo administration of recombinant interleukin-2 induces granulocyte- macrophage colony formation in a murine system. J Biol Response Mod 9:420-425, 1990.

16. Naldini A, Fleischmann WR Jr, Ballas ZK, et al: Interleukin-2 inhibits in vitro granulocyte macrophage colony formation. J Immunol 139:1880-1884, 1987.

17. Fujimori Y, Hara H, Nagai K: Effect of lymphokine-activated killer cell fraction on the development of human hematopoietic progenitor cells. Cancer Res 48: 534-538, 1987.
18. Takahashi M, Oshimi K, Saito H, et al: Inhibition of human granulocyte-macrophage colony formation by interleukin-2 treated lymphocytes. Exp Hematol 16: 226-230, 1988.
19. Savary CA, Lotzova E: Inhibition of human bone marrow and myeloid progenitors by interleukin-2-activated lymphocytes. Exp Hematol 18: 1083-1089, 1990.
20. Nagler A, Greenberg PL, Lanier LL, et al: The effects of recombinant interleukin-2-activated natural killer cells on autologous peripheral blood hematopoietic progenitors. J Exp Med 168:47-54, 1988.
21. van den Brink MRM, Voogt PJ, Marijt WAF, et al: Lymphokine-activated killer cells selectively kill tumor cells in bone marrow without compromising bone marrow stem cell function in vitro. Blood 74:354-360, 1989.
22. Charak BS, Malloy B, Agah R, et al: A novel approach to purging of leukemia by activation of bone marrow with interleukin-2. Bone Marrow Transplant 6:193-198, 1990.
23. Spitzer G, Verma DS, Fisher R, et al: The myeloid progenitor cell—its value in predicting hematopoietic recovery after autologous bone marrow transplantation. Blood 55:317-323, 1980.
24. Charak BS, Agah R, Brynes RK, et al: Interleukin-2 (IL-2) and IL-2-activated bone marrow in transplantation: Evaluation from a clinical perspective. Bone Marrow Transplant 9:479-486, 1992.
25. Charak BS, Brynes RK, Groshen S, et al: Bone marrow transplantation with interleukin-2-activated bone marrow followed by interleukin-2 therapy for acute myeloid leukemia in mice. Blood 76: 2187-2190, 1990.
26. Charak BS, Brynes RK, Chogyoji M, et al: Lymphokine activated killer cells in autologous bone marrow transplantation: Evidence against inhibition of engraftment in vivo. Transplantation 54:1008-1013, 1992.
27. Mazumder A, Rosenberg SA: Successful immunotherapy of natural killer-resistant established pulmonary melanoma metastases by the intravenous adoptive transfer of syngeneic lymphocytes activated in vitro by interleukin-2. J Exp Med 159:495-507, 1984.
28. Thompson JA, Peace DJ, Klarnet JP, et al: Eradication of disseminated murine leukemia by treatment with high-dose interleukin-2. J Immunol 137:3675-3680, 1986.

29. Ujiie T: Increased sensitivity of tumor cells to immune defense cells following treatment with antineoplastic agents in vitro. Jpn J Exp Med 59:17-26, 1989.

30. Ackerstein A, Kedar E, Slavin S, et al: Use of recombinant human interleukin-2 in conjunction with syngeneic bone marrow transplantation in mice as a model for control of minimal residual disease in malignant hematologic disorders. Blood 78:1212-1215, 1991.

31. Charak BS, Brynes RK, Katsuda S, et al: Induction of graft versus leukemia effect in bone marrow transplantation: Dosage and time schedule dependency of interleukin-2 therapy. Cancer Res 51:2015-2020, 1991.

32. Charak BS, Choudhary GD, Tefft M, et al: Interleukin-2 in bone marrow transplantation: Preclinical studies. Bone Marrow Transplant 10:103-111, 1992.

33. Gill I, Agah R, Hu E, et al: Synergistic antitumor effects of interleukin-2 and the monoclonal Lym-1 against human Burkitt lymphoma cells in vitro and in vivo. Cancer Res 49:5377-5379, 1989.

34. Higuichi CM, Thompson JA, Cox T, et al: Lymphokine activated killer function following autologous bone marrow transplantation for refractory hematological malignancies. Cancer Res 49:5509-5513, 1989.

35. Blaise D, Olive D, Stoppa AM, et al: Hematologic and immunologic effects of the systemic administration of recombinant interleukin-2 after autologous bone marrow transplantation. Blood 76:1092-1097, 1990.

36. Charak BS, Mazumder A: Absence of correlation between IL-2-induced NK activity and GVL effect in autologous bone marrow transplantation. Proc Am Assoc Cancer Res 33:1953a, 1992.

37. Lotze MT, Matory YL, Ettinghausen SE, et al: In vivo administration of purified human interleukin-2: Half life, immunologic effects, and expansion of peripheral lymphoid cells in vivo with recombinant IL-2. J Immunol 135:2865-2875, 1985.

38. Merluzzi VJ, Welte K, Last-Barney K, et al: Production and response to interleukin-2 in vitro and in vivo after bone marrow transplantation in mice. J Immunol 134:2426-2430, 1985.

39. Sondel PM, Hanks J, Kohler PC, et al: Destruction of autologous human lymphocytes by interleukin-2-activated cytotoxic cells. J Immunol 137:502-511, 1986.

40. Peace DJ, Cheever MA: Toxicity and therapeutic efficacy of high-dose interleukin-2. In vivo infusion of antibody to NK 1.1 atten-

uates toxicity without compromising efficacy against murine leukemia. J Exp Med 169:161-173, 1989.

41. Azuma E, Yamamoto H, Kaplan J: Use of lymphokine-activated killer cells to prevent bone marrow graft rejection and lethal graft vs host disease. J Immunol 143:1524-1529, 1989.

42. Sykes M, Romick ML, Hoyles KA, et al: In vivo administration of interleukin-2 plus T cell depleted syngeneic marrow prevents graft-versus-host disease mortality and permits alloengraftment. J Exp Med 171:645-658, 1990.

43. Heslop HE, Gottlieb DJ, Bianchi ACM, et al: In vivo induction of γ interferon and tumor necrosis factor by interleukin-2 infusion following intensive chemotherapy or autologous bone marrow transplantation. Blood 74:1374-1380, 1989.

44. Charak BS, Agah R, Gray D, et al: Interaction of various cytokines with interleukin-2 in the generation of killer cells from human bone marrow: Application in purging of leukemia. Leuk Res 15:801-810, 1991.

45. Shiloni E, Eisenthal A, Sachs DM, et al: Antibody dependant cellular cytotoxicity mediated by murine lymphocytes activated in recombinant interleukin-2. J Immunol 138:1992-1998, 1987.

46. Kalofonos H, Rowlinson G, Epenetos AA: Enhancement of monoclonal antibody uptake in human colon tumor xenografts following irradiation. Cancer Res 50:159-163, 1990.

47. Adler A, Chervenick PA, Whiteside TL, et al: Interleukin-2 induction of lymphokine-activated killer (LAK) activity in the peripheral blood and bone marrow of acute leukemic patients. I. Feasibility of LAK generation in adult patients with active disease and in remission. Blood 71: 706-716, 1988.

48. Keever CA, Pekle K, Gazzola MV, et al: NK and LAK activities from human bone marrow progenitors. I. The effects of interleukin-2 and interleukin-1. Cell Immunol 126:211-226, 1990.

49. Bianchi A, Gray P, Kornbluth J: High levels of LAK activity induced from the bone marrow of multiple myeloma patients. Blood 78(Suppl 1):451, 1991.

50. Morecki S, Nabet C, Ackerstein A, et al: The effect of in vitro T lymphocyte depletion on generation of IL-2 activated cytotoxic cells. Bone Marrow Transplant 9:269-273, 1991.

51. Foa R, Caretto P, Fierro MT, et al: Interleukin-2 does not promote the in vitro and in vivo proliferation and growth of human acute leukemia cells of myeloid and lymphoid origin. Br J Haematol 75:34-40, 1990.

52. Broxmeyer HE, Williams DE, Lu L, et al: The suppressive influences of human tumor necrosis factors on bone marrow

hematopoietic progenitor cells from normal donors and patients with leukemia: Synergism of tumor necrosis factor and interferon γ. J Immunol 136:4487-4495, 1986.

53. Klingeman H-G, Grigg AP, Wilkie-Boyd K, et al: Treatment with recombinant interferon (α-2B) early after bone marrow transplantation in patients at high risk of relapse. Blood 78:3306-3311, 1991.

54. Cozzolino F, Rubartelli A, Aldinucci D, et al: Interleukin 1 as an autocrine growth factor for acute myeloid leukemia cells. Proc Natl Acad Sci U S A 86:2369-2373, 1989.

55. Coulombel L, Kalousek D, Eaves CJ, et al: Long-term marrow culture reveals chromosomally normal hematopoitic progenitor cells in patients with Philadelphia chromosome-positive chronic myelogenous leukemia. N Engl J Med 308:1493-1498, 1983.

56. Brandwein JM, Laraya P, Dube ID, et al: Studies of long term marrow culture in patients with acute and chronic myeloid leukemia. Exp Hematol 17:587, 1989.Abstract.

57. Udomsakdi C, Eaves CJ, Swolin B, et al: Rapid decline of chronic myeloid leukemic cells in long term culture due to a defect at the leukemic stem cell level. Proc Natl Acad Sci U S A 11:147-154, 1992.

58. Lotzova E, Savary CA: Generation of NK cell activity from human bone marrow. J Immunol 139:279-284, 1987.

59. Verma UN, Bagg A, Brown E, et al: Interleukin-2 activation of human bone marrow in long term cultures: An effective strategy for purging and generation of antitumor cytotoxic effectors. Bone Marrow Transplant. In press.

60. Klingeman H-G, Eaves C, Eaves AC, et al: Transplantation of autologous bone marrow cultured in interleukin-2 to support myeloablative chemotherapy in poor prognosis acute myeloid leukemia (AML). Blood 78:236a, 1991. Abstract.

61. Lionetti FJ, Luscinskas FW, Hunt SM, et al: Factors affecting the stability of cryogenically preserved granulocytes. Cryobiology 17:297-310, 1980.

62. Charak BS, Areman EA, Dickerson SA, et al: A novel approach to immunomodulation of frozen human bone marrow with interleukin- 2 for clinical application. Bone Marrow Transplant 11:147-154, 1993.

63. Glazier A, Tutschka PJ, Farmer ER, et al: Graft-versus-host disease in cyclosporine A treated rats after syngeneic and autologous bone marrow reconstitution. J Exp Med 158:1-8, 1983.

64. Hess AD, Horwitz L, Beschorner WE, et al: Development of graft-versus-host disease-like syndrome in cyclosporine-treated rats

after syngeneic bone marrow transplantation. I. Development of cytotoxic T-lymphocytes with apparent polyclonal anti-Ia specificity, including autoreactivity. J Exp Med 161:718-730, 1985.

65. Shinozawa T, Beschorner WE, Hess AD: The thymus and prolonged administration of cyclosporine. Irreversible immunopathological changes associated with autologous pseudograft-versus-host disease. Transplantation 50:106-111, 1990.

66. Sorokin R, Kimura H, Schroder K, et al: Cyclosporine- induced autoimmunity. Conditions for expressing disease, requirement for intact thymus, and potency estimates of autoimmune lymphocytes in drug-treated rats. J Exp Med 164:1615-1625, 1986.

67. Jenkins MK, Schwartz RN, Pardoll DM: Effects of cyclosporine A on cell development and clonal deletion. Science 241:1655-1658, 1988.

68. Gao EK, Lo D, Cheney R, et al: Abnormal differentiation of thymocytes in mice treated with cyclosporine A. Nature 336:176-179, 1988.

69. Bryson JS, Caywood BE, Kaplan AM: Relationship of cyclosporine A-mediated inhibition of clonal deletion and development of syngeneic graft-versus-host disease. J Immunol 147:391-397, 1991.

70. Geller RB, Esa AH, Beschorner WE, et al: Successful in vitro graft-versus-tumor effect against an Ia-bearing tumor using cyclosporine-induced syngeneic graft-versus-host disease in the rat. Blood 74:1165-1171, 1989.

71. Chow LH, Mosback-Ozmen L, Ryffel, B, et al: Syngeneic graft-versus-host disease induced by cyclosporine-a reappraisal. Transplantation 46(Suppl):107-112, 1988.

72. Bryson JS, Jennings CD, Caywood BE, et al: Strain specificity in the induction of syngeneic graft-versus-host disease in mice. Transplantation 51:911-913, 1991.

73. Charak BS, Agah R, Mazumder A: Synergism of interleukin-2 and cyclosporine A in induction of a graft versus tumor effect without graft versus host disease after syngeneic bone marrow transplantation. Blood 80:179-184, 1992.

74. Hooton JWL, Miller CL, Helgason CD, et al: Development of precytotoxic T cells in cyclosporine suppressed mixed lymphocyte reactions. J Immunol 144:816-823, 1990.

75. North RJ: Cyclophosphamide-facilitated adoptive immunotherapy of an established tumor depends on elimination of tumor-induced suppressor cells. J Exp Med 155:1063-1074, 1982.

76. Nagarkatti M, Kaplan AM: The role of suppressor T-cells in BCNU-mediated rejection of a syngeneic tumor. J Immunol 135:1510-1517, 1985.

77. Charak, BS, Sadowski RM, Mazumder A: Antitumor effect of interferon plus cyclosporine A following chemotherapy for disseminated melanoma. Cancer Res 52:6482-6486, 1992.

78. Slavin S, Ackerstein A, Naparstek E, et al: The graft- versus-leukemia (GVL) phenomenon: Is GVL separable from GVHD? Bone Marrow Transplant 6:155-161, 1990.

79. Brandt SJ, Peters WP, Atwater SK, et al: Effect of recombinant human granulocyte-macrophage colony stimulating factor on hematopoietic reconstitution after high dose chemotherapy and autologous bone marrow transplantation. N Engl J Med 318:869-876, 1988.

80. Nemunaitis J, Singer JW, Buckner CD, et al: Use of recombinant human granulocyte/macrophage colony stimulating factor (rh GM-CSF) following autologous bone marrow transplantation for lymphoid malignancies. Blood 72:834-836, 1988.

81. Metcalf D: The granulocyte-macrophage colony stimulating factor. Science 229:16-22, 1985.

82. Golde DW: Overview of myeloid growth factors. Semin Hematol 27:1-7, 1990.

83. Cannistra SA, Griffin JD: Regulation of the production and function of granulocytes and monocytes. Semin Hematol 25:173-188, 1988.

84. Kushner BH, Cheung NK: GM-CSF enhances 3F8 monoclonal antibody-dependent cellular cytotoxicity against human melanoma and neuroblastoma. Blood 73:1936-1941, 1989.

85. Ho AD, Haas R, Wulf G, et al: Activation of lymphocytes induced by recombinant human granulocyte-macrophage colony- stimulating factor in patients with malignant lymphoma. Blood 75:203-212, 1990.

86. Wing EJ, Magee DM, Whiteside TL, et al: Recombinant human granulocyte/macrophage colony-stimulating factor enhances monocyte cytotoxicity and secretion of tumor necrosis factor and α interferon in cancer patients. Blood 73:643-646, 1989.

87. Grabstein KH, Urdal DL, Turlinski RJ, et al: Induction of macrophage tumoricidal activity by granulocyte-macrophage colony-stimulating factor. Science 232:506-508, 1986.

88. Epenetos AA, Snook D, Durbin H, et al: Limitations of radiolabelled monoclonal antibodies for localization of human neoplasms. Cancer Res 46:3183-3191, 1986.

89. Charak BS, Sadowski RM, Mazumder A: Granulocyte-macrophage colony-stimulating factor in autologous bone marrow transplantation: Augmentation of graft versus tumor effect via antibody dependent cellular cytotoxicity. Leuk and Lymph 9:453-457, 1993.

90. Charak BS, Agah R, Mazumder A: Granulocyte-macrophage colony-stimulating factor-induced antibody dependent cellular cytotoxicity in bone marrow macrophages: Application in bone marrow transplantation. Blood 81:3474-3479, 1993.
91. Le Berthon B, Khawli LA, Alauddin M, et al: Enhanced tumor uptake of macromolecules induced by a novel vasoactive interleukin-2 immunoconjugate. Cancer Res 51:2696-2698, 1991.
92. Puri RK, Travis WD, Rosenberg SA: Decrease in interleukin- 2-induced vascular leakage in the lungs of mice by administration of recombinant interleukin-1 α in vivo. Cancer Res 49:969-976, 1989.

Chapter 3

Autologous Graft-Versus-Host Disease

Richard J. Jones, M.D., Allan D. Hess, Ph.D.

Bone marrow transplantation (BMT) is effective therapy for patients with high-risk hematologic malignancies, and is probably the treatment of choice for patients with these diseases at relapse. Autologous BMT has become an important alternative to allogeneic BMT in these diseases. The results, with these two approaches, in acute leukemia[1-3] and lymphoma[4-7] are now similar, although the causes for failure are different. Autologous BMT has also shown promising preliminary results in drug-responsive solid tumors like breast cancer. High-dose cytotoxic therapy followed by autologous BMT appears to produce the best results published for patients with metastatic breast cancer, with about a 50% complete response rate and a disease-free survival of 10% to 20% at 4 years.[8,9] Relapse is the major cause of failure in autologous transplants, accounting for at least 90% of the failures. Relapse is much less of a problem following allogeneic BMT, although the improved disease control is largely offset by toxicity resulting from graft-versus-host disease (GVHD). The relapse rate is higher following autologous BMT than after allogeneic BMT, because of the absence of the graft-versus-tumor (GVT) effect associated with allogeneic BMT, and infusion of tumor contaminating autologous marrow grafts. Novel strategies that improve the antitumor activity of autologous BMT are therefore needed.

From: Spitzer T, Mazumder A: Immunotherapy and Bone Marrow Transplantation. Armonk, NY, Futura Publishing Co., Inc., © 1995.

Background

GVHD develops in about 30% to 70% of patients undergoing allogeneic BMT and is a major cause of morbidity and mortality in these patients. However, GVHD also produces a clinically significant immunological antitumor effect, above that produced by the preparative regimen, against leukemias and lymphomas.[2,10-14] A similar allogeneic GVT effect against breast cancer and other nonhematologic malignancies does not appear to exist in animal models.[15,16] A likely reason for the absence of an allogeneic GVT effect against nonhematologic malignancies is that nonhematologic malignancies generally have a lower expression of histocompatibility antigens than hematologic malignancies.[17-19] Attempts to prevent GVHD by T-lymphocyte depletion of allogeneic marrow grafts have led to increased relapse rates following allogeneic BMT.[12,13] Therefore, control of GVHD has not significantly improved survival after allogeneic BMT, as the decreased mortality resulting from GVHD is offset by increased relapse rates. Likewise, although autologous or syngeneic BMT avoid the toxicity of GVHD, the GVT effect is also absent; this appears to be a major reason for the higher relapse rates after autologous and syngeneic BMT compared to allogeneic BMT.[2,10]

Although tumor recurrence remains the major cause for failure of autologous BMT, animal models suggest that a 25% to 50% improvement in relapse rate, as would be needed to cure the majority of patients with high-risk hematologic malignancies who now relapse after autologous BMT, probably requires no more than an average of 1 to 2 logs of additional tumor cell kill.[20,21] However, this small amount of additional tumor cell kill likely represents the most drug-resistant population of cells. Furthermore, current cytotoxic preparative regimens for BMT are at or near nonhematologic dose-limiting toxicity, hindering a further increase in the intensity of these preparative regimens. Other approaches for improving the antitumor activity of autologous BMT are therefore needed. Immunological approaches for eradicating tumors should be particularly effective after autologous BMT, as they would be used in a period of minimal residual disease and should be truly noncross-resistant with the cytotoxic therapy.

A syndrome similar to GVHD develops spontaneously in 5% to 10% of patients undergoing autologous or syngeneic BMT.[22-24] This syndrome clinically resembles GVHD, but it is a mild, self- limited disease that generally involves only the skin. Histologic changes of this "autologous GVHD" are also identical to those of allogeneic GVHD. Autologous GVHD was controversial until the development of animal models for the syndrome.[25-27] In these models, GVHD developed in rats or mice treated with cyclosporine (CsA) after syngeneic BMT. CsA-induced GVHD after syngeneic BMT in rats appears to be mediated by autoreactive lymphocytes directed against Class II histocompatibility (HLA-DR or Ia) antigens.[28]

GVHD after syngeneic BMT in animals exhibits antitumor activity, similar to allogeneic GVHD, against tumors that express Ia antigen.[29,30] Since most lymphomas (including Sternberg-Reed cells of Hodgkin's disease) and acute leukemias express Ia antigens,[17] autologous GVHD could potentially produce a clinical immunological antilymphoma and antileukemia effect without increasing posttransplant toxicity. We have found that autologous GVHD can be induced with CsA in patients undergoing autologous BMT.[31] Moreover, our preliminary results suggest that CsA-induced autologous GVHD manifests clinical antitumor activity, and this results in an improved disease-free survival because autologous GVHD does not increase the posttransplant mortality.[32]

Animal Models

Immunological Mechanisms of Syngeneic Graft-Versus-Host Disease

Glazier et al. reported that rats treated with CsA for 30 to 40 days after syngeneic BMT developed a T-lymphocyte dependent autoimmune syndrome 14 to 28 days after discontinuation of the CsA.[25] Early in its course, this syndrome resembles acute GVHD with erythroderma, dermatitis, and histologic lesions indistinguishable from allogeneic GVHD in the skin and liver.[33] This syngeneic GVHD in rats rapidly progresses to a more chronic form of GVHD with its relevant histologic features.[34] This syndrome can also be induced in mice with the use of CsA.[26,27] Both cluster designation (CD)4+ and CD8+ T lymphocytes are required for the full development of syngeneic GVHD.[35] The transfer of large numbers of CD8+ cells from animals with syngeneic GVHD to normal recipients results in only the acute form of syngeneic GVHD, which resolves in the recipients within 2 weeks. The addition of CD4+ T cells from the animals with syngeneic GVHD both augmented the transfer of the acute form of syngeneic GVHD and also allowed progression to the chronic form. The effector T cells of syngeneic GVHD appear to recognize Ia antigen on target cells.[28,36] Moreover, the effector cells appear to recognize a public determinant of Ia since the effector cells are capable of lysing Ia-bearing cells from multiple strains of rats in addition to self.[28]

Several factors have been shown to be essential for the induction of syngeneic GVHD. This syndrome can only be induced in rats that were treated with CsA for a minimum of 28 days.[37] Total body irradiation (TBI), or other regimens that can ablate the lymphohematopoietic system, are generally necessary for the syndrome to be induced,[25,26] although normal, nontransplanted animals may develop syngeneic GVHD if treated with CsA for extended periods of time (over 6 months).[38] An intact thymus that is included within the irradiation field is also required, as shielding the thymus during TBI results in failure to induce the syndrome.[33] Taken together, it appears that ablation of the lymphohematopoietic system is needed to damage the thymus and to eliminate peripheral host autoregulatory mechanisms. The damaged thymus gives rise to the effector cells of syngeneic GVHD. CsA appears to augment the development of autoreactive lymphocytes by blocking mechanisms that delete autoreactive T cells in the thymus.[39]

Antitumor Activity of Syngeneic Graft-Versus-Host Disease

To determine if syngeneic GVHD exhibited antitumor activity, as is seen with allogeneic GVHD, studies were initiated using the CRL1662 myeloma cell line derived from the LouM strain of rat.[29] This tumor was chosen because it expressed Ia antigen. Syngeneic GVHD had previously been reported to show no antileukemia activity against a rat leukemia;[40] however, this leukemia does not express Ia and therefore would not be expected to be a target of syngeneic GVHD. Splenic T cells from LouM rats that developed syngeneic GVHD were able to lyse CRL1662 tumor cells in vitro.[29] Cytolytic activity of the lymphocytes against the tumor cells declined to baseline as the syngeneic GVHD resolved. Lysis of tumor cells was blocked by preincubation of the tumor cells with antibodies specific for Ia antigen but not with antibodies against Class I antigens. The interferons (IFN), both γ and α, have been shown to up-regulate Ia expression on hematologic malignancies.[41,42] Incubation of the tumor cells with γ-IFN increased the tumor cells' expression of Ia antigen, and also enhanced the lysis of the cells by the lymphocytes obtained from rats with syngeneic GVHD.[29] These studies demonstrated that syngeneic GVHD manifested antitumor activity in vitro, and confirmed that the effector cell was a T lymphocyte specific for the Ia antigen.

Syngeneic GVHD also produces antitumor activity in vivo. Syngeneic GVHD in mice will kill L1210 leukemia cells (which also express Class II antigens) in vivo. An advantage of using this leukemia is that it can be used as a model of minimal residual disease, as just one L1210 cell can kill a mouse.[20,43] This allowed us to demonstrate that syngeneic GVHD will actually cure mice injected with small numbers of L1210 cells. It appeared that syngeneic GVHD was able to kill 1 to 2 logs of L1210 cells in vivo. Syngeneic GVHD in rats will also produce antitumor activity in vivo.[30] Syngeneic GVHD results in about a 1 to 2 log kill of CRL1662 myeloma cells injected into rats. Thus, the magnitude of the immunological antitumor activity generated by syngeneic GVHD appears to be similar to that produced by allogeneic GVHD.[21]

Autologous GVHD appeared to have little toxicity in this animal model; therefore, it may be possible to enhance the activity of the syndrome and potentially increase its effectiveness in vivo. Interleukin (IL)-2 should amplify the effector T lymphocytes in this syndrome. In fact, IL-2 markedly exacerbated the clinical autoimmune syndrome in the animals, leading to the death of all the animals treated with CsA and IL-2. Conversely, both γ-IFN[30] and α-IFN enhanced the antitumor effect of syngeneic GVHD by 1 to 2 logs in the rat model, with the cure of about half of the animals given 50 000 tumor cells. The activity of the IFNs appears to be mediated through increasing the expression of Ia antigen on the tumor, as they have no activity on their own in this animal model. Preliminary data suggest that the addition of low dose IL-2 to IFN may even produce a greater enhancement of antitumor activity associated with syngeneic GVHD.

Human Studies

Based on the results of the animal studies, we designed a study to determine whether GVHD could be induced in patients undergoing autologous BMT for hematologic malignancies.[31] We treated five consecutive patients with aggressive non-Hodgkin's lymphoma (NHL) (three patients) and Hodgkin's disease (two patients) in resistant relapse (no longer responsive to conventional salvage therapy) with autologous BMT and CsA. The preparative regimen was busulfan (BU) plus cyclophosphamide (CY) in three patients who had received prior irradiation, and CY plus TBI in the other 2 patients.

CsA was started on the day of BMT and was continued for 28 days at 1 mg/kg per day. Histologically proven grade II GVHD of the skin developed in all five patients at a median of 11 days (range 9 to 13) after BMT, at the time of initial evidence of hematologic recovery. An erythematous maculopapular rash affecting the face, ears, upper trunk, and extremities (palms and soles) developed in all five patients, and affected the entire body of two patients. No patient developed evidence of extracutaneous GVHD. One patient died of fungal sepsis on day 12 after BMT, and the autologous GVHD resolved in 1 to 3 weeks in the other four patients (spontaneously in 2 patients and with corticosteroids in the other 2). The antigenic specificities of cytotoxic lymphocytes from one of the patients were tested in a cell mediated lysis assay. The lymphocytes collected during autologous GVHD were cytotoxic for the patient's own pretransplant lymphocytes and for lymphocytes from a healthy volunteer. The cytotoxicity was blocked by incubating the target cells with anti-Ia monoclonal antibodies. Lymphocytes obtained after resolution of clinical autologous GVHD would no longer react against the patient's own pretransplant lymphocytes or the healthy donor's lymphocytes. As in the animals with syngeneic GVHD, autoreactive lymphocytes recognizing a public epitope of the Ia antigen appear to mediate clinical autologous GVHD. Other groups have now confirmed our clinical results with inducing autologous GVHD, including finding Ia-restricted autoreactive lymphocytes in patients with autologous GVHD.[44,45]

In order to evaluate the potential antitumor activity of autologous GVHD, we have undertaken a phase II trial to study induced autologous GVHD in patients with intermediate or high- grade NHL in sensitive relapse (still responsive to conventional salvage therapy prior to BMT).[32] Although very few of these patients can be cured with conventional salvage therapy, about 40% to 50% of these patients appear to be curable with autologous BMT.[6,7] Nearly all of the failures following autologous BMT are a consequence of relapse. A 1 to 2 log additional tumor cell kill (as is seen with syngeneic GVHD in animals) over that provided by the preparative regimen, would be expected to decrease the relapse rate by about 20% to 25%.[20,21] We have treated over 25 patients on this protocol. About 80% of the patients have developed histologically proven cutaneous GVHD. The majority of the patients developed autologous GVHD during initial hematologic recovery (at a mean of 18 days after BMT), while on the CsA. About a quarter of the patients developed autologous GVHD after stopping the CsA, usually within 2 weeks of stopping the drug. The autologous GVHD resolved without incident in all patients.

Lymphocytes obtained from patients at the time of autologous GVHD showed Ia-restricted autoreactivity. The preliminary results show that relapse rate was 29% in these patients compared to 50% in 34 consecutive historical controls treated similarly but without CsA ($P=0.03$).[32] However, unlike allogeneic BMT where the decreased relapse rate is offset by increased transplant-related mortality, there were no deaths attributable to autologous BMT; there was an event-free survival benefit for the CsA patients (62% compared to 40%, $P=0.05$).

We have also been able to induce GVHD in patients undergoing autologous BMT with 4-hydroperoxycyclophosphamide purging for acute myeloid leukemia (AML), and the initial antileukemia results likewise look promising.[46] CsA will also induce autologous GVHD in patients undergoing autologous BMT for metastatic breast cancer.[47] However, unlike lymphoma and AML patients where 1 mg/kg per day of CsA was sufficient to induce the syndrome, 2.5 mg/kg per day was required to induce the syndrome in the patients with breast cancer. The higher doses of CsA needed to induce autologous GVHD in breast cancer may be the result of less ablation of host immunoregulatory mechanisms by the BMT preparative regimen or previous conventional-dose therapy (see animal studies above). Higher or more prolonged doses of CsA may be able to surmount these immunoregulatory mechanisms, even without doses of cytotoxic therapy that ablate the lymphohematopoietic system.[38]

There did not appear to be an improvement in tumor control in the breast cancer patients developing autologous GVHD with CsA. This is not surprising as, in contrast to most hematologic malignancies, breast cancers usually do not constitutively express Ia antigen.[18,19] However, Ia-expression can be induced in most breast cancers with the use of γ-IFN.[19] Therefore, we have initiated a pilot clinical trial with γ-IFN to augment CsA-induced autologous GVHD in patients undergoing autologous BMT for metastatic breast cancer.[48] Preliminary results suggest that the severity, but not the incidence, of autologous GVHD has been increased in the patients receiving γ-IFN; however, the autologous GVHD remains self-limited. Furthermore, there may be an improved antitumor effect in the patients receiving γ-IFN. We have also begun a pilot clinical trial of α-IFN with CsA in patients with refractory hematologic malignancies undergoing autologous BMT. α-IFN may be as effective in inducing Ia- expression in hematologic malignancies as γ-IFN[41,42] and, in contrast to γ-IFN, produces little up-regulation of Ia expression on normal tissues.[49] It may, therefore, have a greater selective effect than γ-IFN on Ia expression on leukemias and lymphomas compared to normal cells.

Conclusions

CsA-induced autologous GVHD appears to generate immunological antitumor activity that is similar in magnitude to that seen with allogeneic GVHD. However, whereas the beneficial immunological antitumor activity associated with allogeneic BMT is offset by the toxicity of allogeneic GVHD, autologous GVHD appears to improve the disease-free survival because it does not increase posttransplant mortality. Since autologous GVHD is a mild, self-limited disease, it is possible that the antitumor effect associated with this syndrome could be amplified without substantially increasing toxicity. Furthermore, it should be possible to enhance the clinical antitumor activity of autologous GVHD by immunomodulation of either the effector cells that generate the syndrome, the tumor cells, or both. Stimulation of the effector T cells of autologous GVHD should improve their antitumor activity. A number of cytokines, ie, IL-2 and IL-6,[50] stimulate cytotoxic T cells and can induce antitumor activity. The IFNs up-regulate Ia expression on tumor cells and make these cells more sensitive to the cytotoxic effects of the effector T cells of autologous GVHD.[29,30] We have found that both IL-2 and IFN will increase the antitumor effect of CsA-induced syngeneic GVHD in rats, with the combination of IL-2 and IFN producing the greatest beneficial effect.

Although allogeneic BMT does not appear to be useful for solid tumors because of the absence of an allogeneic GVT effect against these diseases,[15,16] autologous GVHD could potentially have activity against solid tumors as well as hematologic malignancies. While only 30% of breast cancer cells express Ia antigen,[18] most can be induced to express Ia after incubations with γ-IFN.[19] We have begun clinical trials to investigate the toxicity and efficacy of the IFNs combined with CsA-induced autologous GVHD in both hematologic malignancies and breast cancer.

References

1. Yeager AM, Kaizer H, Santos GW, et al: Autologous bone marrow transplantation in patients with acute nonlymphocytic leukemia, using ex vivo marrow treatment with 4-hydroperoxy-cyclophosphamide. N Engl J Med 315:141-147, 1986.
2. Kersey JH, Weisdorf D, Nesbit ME, et al: Comparison of autologous and allogeneic bone marrow transplantation for treatment of high-risk refractory acute lymphoblastic leukemia. N Engl J Med 317:461-467, 1987.

3. Sallan SE, Niemeyer CM, Billett AL, et al: Autologous bone marrow transplantation for acute lymphoblastic leukemia. J Clin Oncol 7:1594-1601, 1989.
4. Jones RJ, Piantadosi S, Mann RB, et al: High-dose cytotoxic therapy and bone marrow transplantation for relapsed Hodgkin's disease. J Clin Oncol 8:527-537, 1990.
5. Carella AM, Congiu AM, Gaozza E, et al: High-dose chemotherapy with autologous bone marrow transplantation in 50 advanced resistant Hodgkin's disease patients: An Italian study group report. J Clin Oncol 6:1411-1416, 1988.
6. Philip T, Armitage JO, Spitzer G, et al: High-dose therapy and autologous bone marrow transplantation after failure of conventional chemotherapy in adults with intermediate-grade or high-grade non-Hodgkin's lymphoma. N Engl J Med 316:1493-1498, 1987.
7. Takvorian T, Canellos GP, Ritz J, et al: Prolonged disease-free survival after autologous bone marrow transplantation in patients with non-Hodgkin's lymphoma with a poor prognosis. N Engl J Med 316:1499-1505, 1987.
8. Peters WP, Shpall EJ, Jones RB, et al: High-dose combination alkylating agents with bone marrow support as initial treatment for metastatic breast cancer. J Clin Oncol 6:1368-1376, 1988.
9. Kennedy MJ, Beveridge RA, Rowley SD, et al: High-dose chemotherapy with reinfusion of purged autologous bone marrow following dose-intense induction as initial therapy for metastatic breast cancer. J Natl Cancer Inst 83:920-926, 1991.
10. Weiden PL, Flournoy N, Thomas ED, et al: Antileukemic effect of graft-versus-host disease in human recipients of allogeneic-marrow grafts. N Engl J Med 300:1068-1073, 1979.
11. Weiden PL, Sullivan KM, Flournoy N, et al: Antileukemic effect of chronic graft-versus-host disease. N Engl J Med 304:1529-1533, 1981.
12. Butturini A, Bortin MM, Gale RP: Graft-versus-leukemia following bone marrow transplantation. Bone Marrow Transplant 2:233-242, 1987.
13. Horowitz MM, Gale RP, Sondel PM, et al: Graft-versus-leukemia reactions after bone marrow transplantation. Blood 75:555-562, 1990.
14. Jones RJ, Ambinder RF, Piantadosi S, et al: Evidence of a graft-versus-lymphoma effect associated with allogeneic bone marrow transplantation. Blood 77:649-653, 1991.
15. Santos GW: Effect of graft-versus-host disease on a spontaneous adenocarcinoma in mice. Exp Hematol 20:46-48, 1970.

16. Fefer A: Immunotherapy of primary Moloney sarcoma virus-induced tumors. Int J Cancer 5:327-332, 1970.
17. Foon KA, Todd RF III: Immunologic classification of leukemia and lymphoma. Blood 68:1-31, 1986.
18. Zuk JA, Walker RA: HLA class II sublocus expression in benign and malignant breast epithelium. J Pathol 155:301-309, 1988.
19. Gastl G, Marth C, Leiter E, et al: Effects of human recombinant α_2 arg-interferon and γ-interferon on human breast cancer cell lines: Dissociation of antiproliferative activity and induction of HLA-DR antigen expression. Cancer Res 45:2957-2961, 1985.
20. Skipper HE, Schabel FM Jr, Wilcox WS: Experimental evaluation of potential anticancer agents. XIII. On the criteria and kinetics associated with "curability" of experimental leukemia. Cancer Chemother Rep 35:1-111, 1964.
21. Hageenbeek A, Martens ACM, Schultz FW: The graft-versus-leukemia reaction after allogeneic bone marrow transplantation only adds one log of leukemia cell kill. Blood 72:390a, 1988. Abstract.
22. Rappeport J, Mihm M, Reinherz E, et al: Acute graft-versus-host disease in recipients of bone-marrow transplants from identical twin donors. Lancet 2:717-720, 1979.
23. Hood AF, Vogelsang GB, Black LP, et al: Acute graft-vs-host disease. Development following autologous and syngeneic bone marrow transplantation. Arch Dermatol 123:745-750, 1987.
24. Einsele H, Ehninger G, Schneider EM, et al: High frequency of graft-versus-host like syndromes following syngeneic bone marrow transplantation. Transplantation 45:579-585, 1988.
25. Glazier A, Tutschka PJ, Farmer ER, et al: Graft-versus-host disease in cyclosporin A-treated rats after syngeneic and autologous bone marrow reconstitution. J Exp Med 158:1-8, 1983.
26. Cheney RT, Sprent J: Capacity of cyclosporine to induce auto-graft-versus-host disease and impair intrathymic T cell differentiation. Transplant Proc 17:528-530, 1985.
27. Bryson JS, Jennings CD, Caywood BE, et al: Induction of a syngeneic graft-versus-host disease like syndrome in DBA/2 mice. Transplantation 48:1042-1047, 1989.
28. Hess AD, Horwitz L, Beschorner WE, et al: Development of graft-vs-host disease like syndrome in cyclosporine-treated rats after syngeneic bone marrow transplantation. J Exp Med 161:718-730, 1985.
29. Geller RB, Esa AH, Beschorner WE, et al: Successful in vitro graft-versus-tumor effect against an Ia-bearing tumor using cy-

closporine-induced syngeneic graft-versus-host disease in the rat. Blood 74:1165-1171, 1989.

30. Noga SJ, Horwitz L, Kim H, et al: Interferon-γ potentiates the antitumor effect of cyclosporine-induced autoimmunity. J Hematotherapy 1:75-84, 1992.

31. Jones RJ, Vogelsang GB, Hess AD, et al: Induction of graft-versus-host disease after autologous bone marrow transplantation. Lancet 1:754-757, 1989.

32. Jones RJ, Vogelsang GB, Ambinder RF, et al: Autologous marrow transplantation (ABMT) with cyclosporine (CSA)-induced autologous graft-versus-host disease (GVHD) for relapsed aggressive non-Hodgkin's lymphoma (NHL). Blood 78:287a, 1991. Abstract.

33. Glazier A, Tutschka PJ, Farmer ER: Studies on the immunobiology of syngeneic and autologous graft-versus-host disease in cyclosporine treated rats. Transplant Proc 15:3035, 1983.

34. Beschorner WE, Shinn CA, Fischer AC, et al: Cyclosporine-induced pseudo-graft-versus-host disease in the early post-cyclosporine period. Transplantation 46:112-117, 1988.

35. Hess AD, Fischer AC, Beschorner WE: Effector mechanisms in cyclopsorine A-induced syngeneic graft-versus-host disease: Role of CD4+ and CD8+ T lymphocyte subsets. J Immunol 145:526-533, 1990.

36. Sorokin R, Kimura H, Schroder K, et al: Cyclosporine-induced autoimmunity: Conditions for expressing disease, requirement for intact thymus, and potency estimates of autoimmune lymphocytes in drug-treated rats. J Exp Med 164:1615, 1986.

37. Hess AD, Fischer AC: Immune mechanisms in cyclosporine-induced syngeneic graft-versus-host disease. Transplantation 48:895-900, 1989.

38. Shinozowa T, Beschorner WE, Hess AD: Prolonged administration of cyclosporine and the thymus: Irreversible immunopathologic changes associated with autologous pseudo-graft-versus-host disease. Transplantation 50:106-111, 1990.

39. Jenkins MK, Schwartz RH, Pardoll DM: Effects of cyclosporine A on T cell development and clonal deletion. Science 241:1655-1658, 1988.

40. Tutschka PJ, Berkowitz SD, Tuttle S, et al: Graft-versus-leukemia in the rat—the antileukemic efficacy of syngeneic and allogeneic graft-versus-host disease. Transplant Proc XIX:2668-2673, 1987.

41. Baldini L, Cortelezzi A, Polli N, et al: Human recombinant interferon α-2C enhances the expression of class II HLA antigens on hairy cells. Blood 67:458-464, 1986.

42. Gressier VH, Weinkauff RE, Franklin WA, et al: Modulation of the expression of major histocompatibility antigens on splenic hairy cells—differential effect upon in vitro treatment with alpha-2b-interferon, gamma-interferon, and interleukin-2. Blood 72:1048-1053, 1988.
43. Jones RJ, Colvin OM, Sensenbrenner LL: Prediction of the ability to purge tumor from murine bone marrow using clonogenic assays. Cancer Res 48:3394-3397, 1988.
44. Dale BM, Atkinson K, Kotasek D, et al: Cyclosporine-induced graft vs host disease in two patients receiving syngeneic bone marrow transplants. Transplant Proc 21:3816-3817, 1989.
45. Carella AM, Gaozza E, Congiu A, et al: Cyclosporine-induced graft-versus-host disease after autologous bone marrow transplantation in hematological malignancies. Ann Hematol 62:156-159, 1991.
46. Yeager AM, Vogelsang GB, Jones RJ, et al: Induction of cutaneous graft-versus-host disease by administration of cyclosporine to patients undergoing autologous bone marrow transplantation for acute myeloid leukemia. Blood 79:3031-3035, 1992.
47. Kennedy MJ, Vogelsang GB, Beveridge RA, et al: Phase I trial of intravenous cyclosporine to induce graft-versus-host disease in women undergoing autologous bone marrow transplantation for breast cancer. J Clin Oncol 11:478-484, 1993.
48. Kennedy MJ, Vogelsang GB, Morris L, et al: Phase I study of gamma-interferon (IFN) to augment cyclosporine A (CSA) induced autologous graft versus host disease (AGVHD) following high-dose chemotherapy (HDC) with autologous marrow reinfusion (AMR) for metastatic breast cancer (MBC). Proc Am Soc Clin Oncol 11:49, 1992. Abstract.
49. Basham T, Smith W, Lanier L, et al: Regulation of expression of class II major histocompatibility antigens on human peripheral blood monocytes and langerhans cells by interferon. Hum Immunol 10:83-93, 1984.
50. Mule JJ, McIntosh JK, Jablons DM, et al: Antitumor activity of recombinant Interleukin 6 in mice. J Exp Med 171:629-636, 1990.

Chapter 4

Monoclonal Antibody Serotherapy as Adjuvant Therapy after Bone Marrow Transplant or Chemotherapy for Malignant Diseases

Edward D. Ball, M.D., Kathy J. Selvaggi, M.D.

High dose chemotherapy supported by bone marrow (BM) or peripheral blood stem cell transplantation for malignant disorders has become a standard treatment in many situations. Patients with leukemia, (acute myeloid, lymphoid and chronic myeloid) and patients with malignant lymphoma (ML) or Hodgkin's disease who have failed initial therapy can be cured by autologous or allogeneic bone marrow transplantation (BMT). In addition, high-dose chemotherapy and autologous BM or peripheral blood stem cell support is increasingly used to treat advanced stage or poor prognosis breast cancer. In all of these diseases, relapse is still a major problem limiting the curative potential of the procedure. Presumably, the principal reason for relapse is failure of the preparative regimen to eradicate all disease in the patient. Since the doses of chemotherapeutic agents are already at the limits of extra-medullary toxicity, it is unlikely that improved disease control will come from further ma-

From: Spitzer T, Mazumder A: Immunotherapy and Bone Marrow Transplantation. Armonk, NY, Futura Publishing Co., Inc., © 1995.

nipulations of currently used ablative regimens. Thus, an alternative approach is to increase in vivo cell kill through other mechanisms such as immunologically mediated cytoreduction. This chapter will focus on the possible role of humoral immune reactions mediated by passive immunotherapy with monoclonal antibodies (MAB). We will first briefly review the potential target molecules for immunotherapy. The reader is referred to more comprehensive reviews of cell surface markers that have been published recently.[1] We will then describe the mechanisms of immunotherapy possible with MAB, and review the clinical trials in progress.

Tumor-Associated Antigens on Myeloid, Lymphoid, and Breast Carcinoma Cells

A large number of murine MABs, reactive with differentiation antigens present on human leukocytes (myeloid and lymphoid) and epithelial cells, have been produced over the past decade (Table 1).[1-3] Malignant cells from patients with acute myeloid leukemia (AML) and acute lymphoblastic leukemia (ALL) and breast carcinoma cells also express these antigens.[1,2]

Table 1
Antigenic Targets for Serotherapy of Minimal Residual Disease in Malignancy

	Myeloid Leukemia	Lymphoid Leukemia	Lymphoma, B cell	Breast Carcinoma
Monoclonal antibody	PM-81 My9 M195	B4	B4	PM-81, BcA 200
Antigen	Le-x, gp67	gp95	gp95	Le-x, her-2/NEU
Cluster designation	15, 33	19	19	15
Normal tissue distribution	PMNs[1] Mono[2]	B cells	B cells	PMNs, Mono

[1] PMN=polymorphonuclear leukocyte
[2] Mono=monocyte

Myeloid Antigens

The series of human leukocyte antigen workshops have delineated a number of cell surface antigens commonly expressed on normal myeloid cells that are also expressed on myeloid leukemia cells. These include cluster designation (CD)11b, CD13, CD14, CD15, CD16, CD33, and CD64.[2] Many of the myeloid surface antigens are expressed commonly on leukemia cells from patients with AML.[2] In fact, the relative state of differentiation of myeloid leukemia cells can be inferred from the degree of expression of lineage-restricted antigens whose emergence during normal myeloid differentiation has been mapped. Certain antigens emerge early, particularly CD33.[4] Others emerge at the level of differentiation characteristic of the normal colony forming unit-granulocyte macrophage (CFU-GM) such as CD13, and CD15. Others appear later and are highly expressed on mature myeloid cells (CD11b, CD14, and CD64). In addition, several groups have examined the cell surface phenotype of clonogenic leukemia cells (L-CFC), the putative leukemic stem cells.[5] These studies have revealed that discrete patterns of both myeloid and lymphoid L-CFC phenotype exist, suggesting that limited maturation of the leukemic clone occurs in association with changes in cell surface antigens in a manner analogous to the patterns of antigen expression of normal colony forming unit-culture (CFU-C). L-CFC from some cases of AML express a relatively immature phenotype, while the majority of cases demonstrate a more differentiated antigenic phenotype that is similar to the CFU-GM.[5]

Some AML-associated antigens are expressed to a greater degree on the L-CFC than their progeny AML-1-99, (no CD),[6] CD33[5] while others are expressed on both populations (CD15),[6] and some are expressed more on the more mature cells of the clone (CD11b).[5] Interpretation of studies using MAB to characterize L-CFC are highly dependent on the MAB used. There are differences in binding avidity and the ability to mediate cytotoxicity.

Several MAB have either been used preclinically or clinically for BM purging for autologous transplantation. These include PM-81 (anti-CD15),[7] AML-2-23 (anti-CD14),[8] CF-1 (anti-CD38) (Reading), S4-7 (anti-CD15),[9] M195 (anti-CD33),[10] My9 (anti-CD33)[11]

Lymphoid Antigens

Normal B and T lymphocytes express a repertoire of cell surface antigens defined by MAB. As in myeloid leukemia, lymphoblastic leukemias and MLs also express these antigens in a differentiation-dependent manner. Murine MAB to human differentiation antigens CD24, CD9 (p-24), CD10, common acute lymphoid leukemia antigen (CALLA), and CD19 bind to common variant ALL and B-lineage ALL, while antibodies to CD5 and CD7 react with T-lineage ALL (Table 1).

Breast Carcinoma-Associated Antigens

Since high-dose chemotherapy with autologous stem cell rescue for metastatic breast cancer is increasingly in use, this is another treatment area that might benefit from adjuvant approaches to eliminating residual disease. There are numerous breast cancer-associated antigens that can be targeted.[3,12,13]

Effector Mechanisms for Monoclonal Antibodies

The efficacy of a MAB-based therapy is dependent on the ability of the MAB to mediate killing of malignant target cells. The process of binding to the cell surface molecule will not usually result in cell death unless an effector mechanism is called upon. Some of the most likely methods to be used are reviewed below.

Complement

The complement (C) system is one means by which cytolysis can be achieved. Murine antibodies of the Ig(Immunoglobulin)G2a, IgG2b, and IgM generally activate C when bound to target cells that express a cell surface antigen in sufficient density. Murine MAB of the IgG1 subclass do not fix C. Murine MAB of the IgM class are capable of activating human C.[14] Thus, human serum or plasma can also serve as a source of C and in vivo serotherapy that depends on endogenous C is feasible.

In order to develop therapeutic reagents that might not be as immunogenic as murine MAB, some investigators have begun to chimerize MAB using genetic engineering technology. It is possible to clone into a human IgG1 genetic construct the unique CDR (Cluster Designation Region) of a murine MAB.[15-20] Thus, the resulting antibody molecule will be primarily "human" with only the unique amino acids of the murine MAB contributing to the binding site. The advantage of such a molecule is that it should be less immunogenic, will retain the unique binding characteristics of the murine MAB, and be able to recruit the effector mechanisms for cytolysis (C activation and antibody-dependent cytotoxicity).

Antibody-Dependent Cellular Cytotoxicity

The Fc fragment of an IgG antibody molecule can bind to one or more of the family of Fc receptors (FcgR I, II, and III). Effector cells expressing these molecules are thus recruited to bind to target cells expressing the antigen to which the Fab portion of the antibody is directed and activated by the cross-linking of adjacent receptor molecules. The result is the delivery of cytotoxic signals to target cells that result in lysis or cell death by other mechanisms. Murine MAB of the IgG2a and IgG3 subclasses are capable of interacting with the type I FcgR, while IgG1 and IgG2b do not react with FcgR1. All classes of IgG interact with the type II and III FcgR when presented in the aggregated form. Receptors for IgM are not believed to exist.

Anti-tumor antibodies alone can thus mediate antibody-dependent cellular cytotoxicity (ADCC) if they can interact with one or more of the FcgR. A novel approach to augmenting ADCC is through the creation of bispecific antibodies comprised of an antitumor MAB and an antibody directed to one of the FcgR, or alternatively, the CD3 molecule on T cells. Such approaches are currently under development and have been introduced into clinical trials (see below).

Immunotoxins

MAb can be coupled to toxins such as ricin, forming immunotoxins (IT). The toxin molecules are lectins derived from plants and consist of two chains, A and B. The A chain is the active agent that can irreversibly inactivate the 60S subunit of ribosomes and inhibit protein synthesis. The B chain mediates uptake into the cell by binding to galactose residues on glycoproteins of the cell membrane. ITs have been constructed either with the whole toxin molecule or with the A chain only, in an attempt to limit toxicity.[21]

Roy et al. have prepared an IT comprised of the My9 MAB and a "blocked" ricin molecule, chemically modified to limit nonspecific uptake via galactose residues.[22] Nadler et al. have developed an IT to B cells using the B4 (anti-CD19) MAB coupled to a modified ricin molecule.[23] This IT is now in clinical trial as a post-BMT adjuvant for patients with non-Hodgkin's lymphoma (see below).

Radionuclides

Another approach to enhancing MAB mediated toxicity against tumors is to couple the MAB to radionuclides that are cytotoxic. Common reagents include Yttrium-90, Iodine-131 (^{131}I), and Rhenium 186 or 188.[24] The advantage of radiolabeled MAB is that antigen negative cells residing near antigen positive cells will also be killed if the appropriate isotope is used. The disadvantage of these reagents is their nonspecific toxicity to other cells encountered in the circulation and the reticuloendothelial system, and the difficulty of delivering therapy with radioactive compounds.

Potential Limitations of
Monoclonal Antibody Serotherapy

Despite the therapeutic promise of tumor-specific or selective reagents such as MABs, there are some obstacles to successful therapy that need to be overcome. These include antigen-negative cells that will not be killed by MAB. This obstacle is overcome by radiolabeled MAB. For other MAB approaches, the possibility that some cells will escape the killing mechanism is real. However, it is theoretically possible that small numbers of tumor cells can be eliminated by natural killing mechanisms. At this time, it is not known how many tumor cells can be allowed to escape without relapse being inevitable. Some antigens "modulate," meaning that the antibody induces patching, capping and endocytosis of the cell surface antigens. This process renders the cell's surface antigen negative. There may be difficulties with delivery of MAB to all sites of disease due to poor vascularization of tumors, especially large solid tumor masses. There may be circulating antigens that can block the binding of MAB to tumor cells. There may be normal cells expressing the antigen that can act as "cold targets" and that might contribute to toxicity of the MAB by either the loss of function of these cells or by release of cellular contents. Finally, when using murine MAB, there may be an immune response to the foreign protein resulting in the neutralization of the MAB. This can be overcome by using humanized MAB.[23,25,26]

In addition, serotherapy with MAB also has a variety of potential adverse reactions, including rigors, pruritus, urticaria and bronchospasm. In many studies, these are seen in less than one third of patients[27] Anaphylaxis has rarely occurred.

Current Status of Autologous and Allogeneic Bone Marrow Transplantation in Acute Myeloid Leukemia, Acute Lymphoblastic Leukemia, Lymphoma (Non-Hodgkin's and Hodgkin's), and Breast Cancer

BMT for patients with leukemias, lymphomas, and certain solid tumors can successfully prolong disease-free intervals and cure a certain proportion of patients. The limitations of BMT are procedure-related complications such as infections, organ toxicities, graft-versus-host disease (GVHD) and relapse of the primary malignant disease. Relapse following high-dose chemotherapy occurs in 25% to 50% of patients with AML and ALL in first or second remission, 50% of patients with lymphoma undergoing BMT after failing initial therapy, and 50% to 80% of patients with breast cancer. Relapses occur because of a failure of high-dose therapy to eradicate all disease from within the patient, a failure of graft-versus-tumor (GVT) effects in allogeneic BMT, and possibly from reintroduction in the marrow graft in autologous BMT. Thus, current clinical trials are beginning to address the issue of residual disease remaining in the patient by designing interventions that can kill the few remaining tumor cells after BMT. These approaches include immunotherapy as well as chemotherapy. Immunotherapy can include the use of cellular therapy with natural killer cells along with interleukins (IL), as well as MAB used either in an unconjugated form taking advantage of natural effector functions such as ADCC and C activation or conjugated to toxins or radionuclides.

Clinical Trials of Monoclonal Antibody Serotherapy

Many Phase I trials of hematologic malignancies using in vivo infusions of MABs directed at antigens on the surface of tumor cells have been completed.[5,16,28-33] Rapid antibody-mediated clearance of tumor cells and occasional complete remissions were demonstrated.[30] In the majority of trials, MABs were delivered by intravenous infusion over several hours. In addition, almost all patients on these trials were refractory to prior chemotherapeutic and radiotherapeutic regimens. Responses have been limited by several problems, including delivery of MAB to the antigen-bearing cells, poor vascularization of tumors, short half-lives of murine immunoglobulins (Ig) in the plasma, the development of blocking antigen in the host, host reaction to murine Igs, shedding of cell-surface antigens, and antigenic modulation which involves internalization or sloughing of the antigen in response to binding by the antibody.[23,25,26] Human anti-mouse antibody (HAMA) responses have occurred in patients receiving MAB therapy. The development of HAMA could potentially decrease the effects of the MAB, presumably due to enhanced clearance of the antibody from the circulation, the formation of antigen-antibody complexes with possible end-organ damage, or the neutralization of the antibody's effects. Studies are now underway using genetically restructured antibodies in which rodent variable or hypervariable Ig regions are combined with human Ig genes to minimize the antigenic determinants.[16,34]

As previously stated, if a MAB is to work in vivo, it must be able to activate C, or mediate ADCC for it to kill tumor cells. The CAM-PATH-1 IgG2b antibody has been used for serotherapy because it both fixes human C and is active in ADCC. Although responses to this antibody were transient, reductions in the circulating malignant lymphocytes were seen.[35]

Studies using anti-idiotype antibodies against B-cell malignancies are ongoing and responses have been observed.[36] Due to shared idiotypes common to many tumors, the need to produce unique idiotype-specific antibody for each patient's tumor is unnecessary; however, idiotype negative clones of cells have been identified.[37-39] As a result, malignant cells can escape this form of therapy.

Some studies have targeted MABs against growth receptors on the surface malignant cells. The anti-Tac MAB is directed against the IL-2 receptor whose function may be integral for tumor proliferation.[40] Three complete and three partial responses in patients with adult T-cell leukemia/lymphoma receiving serotherapy with the anti-Tac MAB has been reported.[41]

A panel of cytotoxic MABs have been described that react specifically with myeloid cells and that recognize antigens expressed on AML blast cells.[2] PM-81 (anti-CD15) is reactive with leukemia cells from >90% of patients with AML.[7] It is reactive with leukemia-colony forming cells (L-CFC) and this reactivity can be predicted by flow cytometry. Although studies have revealed that PM-81 recognizes antigens present of some normal myeloid progenitors, the antibody does not bind to pluripotent stem cells. PM-81, an IgM MAB, is cytotoxic to AML cells in the presence of human C and therefore is cytotoxic to early malignant myeloid leukemia precursors, without toxicity to normal hematopoietic stem cells.

PM-81 is produced by a hybridoma cell line derived from the chemically induced polyethylene glycol fusion of the mouse P3-NS1-1Ag4 (N1) myeloma cell line in spleen cells from a female BALB/c mouse sensitized with peripheral leukemic granulocytes/monocytes from a patient with AML.

A limited Phase I clinical trial has been conducted in which four terminally ill AML patients with resistant disease in relapse were treated with PM-81 in vivo.[42] The MAB was given by slow intravenous infusion diluted in normal saline in doses as high as 210 mg over 24 hours and 600 mg in 7 days. In all cases, circulating leukemic blast counts decreased to levels approximately 25% of the pretreatment levels. However, the effects on circulating blasts were transient. Toxicity was minor and limited; two patients experienced minor back pain and myalgias, which diminished with a slower rate in infusion. A transient decrease in circulating neutrophils was also observed. The mechanism of leukemia cell removal from the circulation was presumed to be cytolysis, since the depression of peripheral blood neutrophils and blast counts occurred concomitantly with a rise in leukocyte lactate dehydrogenase (LDH) isoenzymes during treatment.

The exact mechanism of cytolysis is unclear. IgM MAB mediated cytolysis may occur through the fixation of C3b to C receptors on phagocytic cells in the absence of activation of the subsequent C components. Also, the IgM MAB binds to normal phagocytic cells, as well as leukemia cells, and may have acted as bridges between the target and effector cells without the participation of C or Fc receptors. Insight into the mechanism of IgM mediated cytotoxicity comes from a study by Wagner et al. using a murine MAB directed to a rat leukemia-associated antigen.[43] In this study, the investigators performed BMTs on brown Norway rats that had been inoculated with syngeneic leukemia cells prior to BMT. The rats were then treated intraperitoneally with either control MAB or the IgM MAB directed to an antigen expressed on the leukemia cells. The specific MAB-treated rats experienced a 60% cure rate while the controls all died of leukemia. The doses used were 3 mg/kg body weight. C dependence was shown by depleting endogenous C with cobra venom factor which abrogated the efficacy of MAB.

As an adjunct to standard chemotherapy for patients with relapsed AML or secondary leukemias, we are currently evaluating the role of in vivo MAB therapy (Figure 1). Patients will receive the PM-81 MAB intravenously over 24 hours followed by induction

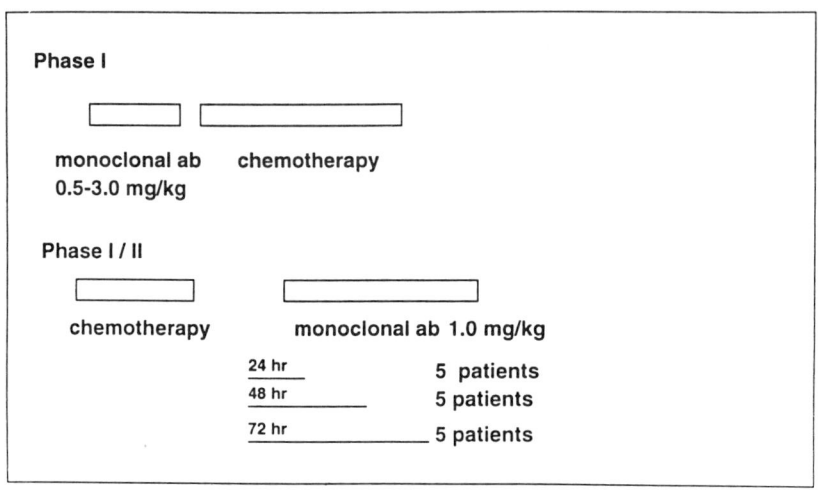

Figure 1. Clinical trials of PM-81 MAB-mediated therapy for AML.

chemotherapy. This current Phase I study objectives are to determine the safety of PM-81 administration in patients with AML, to determine the rate of clearance of circulating MAB dose and percent reduction in circulating blast count, and to determine the possible mechanisms of blast cell cytolysis by measuring C levels, LDH isoenzymes, and percentage of free and cell-bound MAB. Phase I/II trials will be initiated, in which the MAB will be administered postchemotherapy at the time of aplasia when there will be fewer competing cells and the MAB will be treating only minimal residual disease. Five patients will receive MAB 1 mg/kg over 24 hours for 1 day. Five additional patients will receive 1 mg/kg over 24 hours for 2 days, and then a third cohort of five patients will be treated at 1 mg/kg every 24 hours for 3 days. It is perhaps a combination of new modalities as well as existing therapies that will lead to a curative approach for hematologic malignancies.

As mentioned previously, the challenge in treating AML with MABs is the necessity to select an antigen target which is found on the clonogenic myeloid leukemia blast cells, but not on the normal hematopoietic progenitors. Scheinberg et al. recently reported a Phase I trial of MAB M195 in AML.[44] M195 is a mouse IgG 2A reactive with CD33 that is capable of rapidly internalizing into target cells after binding. It is unable to kill cells in vitro by use of human C or effector cells. Other than committed hematopoietic progenitor cells and some monocytes, M195 does not appear to react with any normal cells or tissues.[33,45] This study was designed to answer the following questions: Could an antibody that binds to CD33 be administered safely? Would the binding by a noncytotoxic murine antibody alone result in biological responses, toxicity, or regression? What are the pharmacokinetics, localization, characteristics used to design trials in which M195 is used as a carrier of a cytotoxic isotope or other agent? Their preliminary data indicated that whole BM ablative doses of [131]Iodine (^{131}I)-M195 could be expected. However, tumor regressions were not observed in this study.

Appelbaum et al. are also using an ^{131}I radio labeled anti-CD33 MAB (p67) as part of a marrow transplant preparative regimen for AML.[24] Four patients received 110 to 330 mCi ^{131}I conjugated to p67 followed by a standard transplant regimen of cyclophosphamide plus 12 Gy total body irradiation (TBI). All of them tolerated the procedure and are alive in remission 6.5 to 16 months posttransplant.

Recently, Grossbard et al. studied the IT, anti-B4-blocked ricin. This MAB is directed against B-lineage-restricted CD19 antigen expressed on more than 95% of normal and neoplastic B cells.[23] A Phase I dose escalation clinical trial was conducted in 25 patients with refractory B-cell malignancies. The MAB was administered by daily 1-hour bolus infusions for 5 consecutive days, with doses ranging from 1 mcg/kg per day to 60 mcg/kg per day. The maximum tolerated dose was determined to be 50 mcg/kg per day for 5 days, for a total dose of 250 mcg/kg. The dose limiting toxicity was defined by transient reversible Grade 3 elevations in hepatic transaminases without impaired hepatic synthetic function. One complete response, two partial responses, and eight mixed, or transient, responses were observed, revealing the in vitro and in vivo cytotoxicity of the anti-B4-bR and indicate that this IT can be administered safely as a daily bolus infusion for 5 days. There is now a Phase III Cancer and Leukemia Group B trial of the use of B4-ricin following BMT for ML.

Conclusions

The application of MAB therapy to the treatment of minimal residual disease is in the very early stages of clinical investigation. Phase I and II studies are promising, as are animal models. Since the maximal benefit of high-dose chemotherapy seems to have been reached with currently available agents, new approaches to the control of malignant diseases are needed. Immunological manipulations represent a new approach to achieving a greater degree of cell kill with the promise of decreasing relapses after currently available therapy. Clearly, a number of years will pass before the value of the approaches reviewed in this chapter will be demonstrated.

References

1. Vaickus L, Ball E, Foon K: Immune markers in hematologic malignancies. Crit Rev Oncol/Hematol 11:267, 1991.
2. Ball E: Immunophenotyping of acute myeloid leukemia cells. Clin Lab Med 10:721, 1990.
3. Tjandra JJ, McKenzie IFC: Murine monoclonal antibodies in breast cancer: An overview. Br J Surg 75:1067, 1988.
4. Griffin JD, Lynch D, Sabbath K, et al: A monoclonal antibody reactive with normal and leukemic human myeloid progenitor cells. Leuk Res 4:521, 1984.
5. Sabbath KD, Ball ED, Larcom P, et al: Heterogeneity of clonogenic cells in acute myeloblastic leukemia assessed by surface marker analysis. J Clin Invest 75:746, 1985.
6. Howell A, Stukel T, Bloomfield C, et al: Induction of Differentiation in blast cells and leukemia colony-forming cells (L-CFC) from patients with acute myeloid leukemia. Blood 75:721, 1990.
7. Ball E, Graziano R, Fanger M: A unique antigen expressed on myeloid cells and acute leukemia blast cells defined by a monoclonal antibody. J Immunol 130:2937, 1983.
8. Ball ED, Graziano RF, Shen L, et al: Monoclonal antibodies to novel myeloid antigens reveal human neutrophil heterogeneity. Proc Natl Acad Sci U S A 79:5374, 1982.
9. DeFabritiis P, Ferrero D, Sandrelli A, et al: Monoclonal antibody purging and autologous bone marrow transplantation in acute myelogenous leukemia in complete remission. Bone Marrow Transplant 4:669, 1989.
10. Lemoli R, Gasparetto C, Scheinberg D, et al: Autologous bone marrow transplantation in acute myelogenous leukemia: In vitro treatment with myeloid-specific monoclonal antibodies and drugs in combination. Blood 77:1829, 1991.
11. Robertson MJ, Soiffer RJ, Freedman AS, et al: Human bone marrow depleted of CD33-positive cells mediates delayed but durable reconstitution of hematopoiesis: Clinical trial of MY9 monoclonal antibody-purged autografts for the treatment of acute myeloid leukemia. Blood 79(9):2229, 1992.
12. Ring DB, Clark R, Saxena A: Identity of BCA200 and c-erbB-2 indicated by reactivity of monoclonal antibodies with recombinant c-erbB-2. Mol Immunol 28(8):915, 1992.
13. Frankel AE, Ring DB, Tringale F, et al: Tissue distribution of breast cancer-associated antigens defined by monoclonal antibodies. J Biol Response Mod 4:273, 1984.
14. Ball ED, Guyre PM, Bodwell J, et al: Re-directed killing of HL-

60 Leukemia Cells by gamma interferon activated monocytes using bispecific antibodies to CD15 and the high affinity IgG Fc receptor, FcgRI. Blood 74 (Suppl 1):19, 1989.

15. Winter G, Milstein C: Man-made antibodies. Nature 349:293, 1991.

16. Hale G, Clarke R, Marcus G, et al: Remission induction in non-Hodgkins' lymphoma with reshaped human monoclonal antibody CAMPATH-1H. Lancet 2:1394, 1988.

17. Gorman SD, Clark MR, Routledge EG, et al: Reshaping a therapeutic CD4 antibody. Proc Natl Acad Sci U S A 8:4181, 1991.

18. Queen C, Schneider WP, Selick HE, et al: A humanized antibody than binds to the interleukin 2 receptor. Proc Natl Acad Sci U S A 86:10029, 1989.

19. Co MS, Deschamps M, Whitley RJ, et al: Humanized antibodies for antiviral therapy. Proc Natl Acad Sci U S A 88:2869, 1991.

20. Co MS, Avdalovic NM, Caron PC, et al: Chimeric and humanized antibodies with specificity for the CD33 antigen. J Immunol 148:1149, 1991.

21. Vallera D, Ash R, Zanjani E, et al: Anti-T-cell reagents for human bone marrow transplantation: Ricin linked to three monoclonal antibodies. Science 222:512, 1985.

22. Roy D, Griffin J, Belvin M, et al: Anti-My9-blocked ricin: An immunotoxin for selective targeting of acute myeloid leukemia cells. Blood 77:2404, 1991.

23. Grossbard ML, Freedman AS, Ritz J, et al: Serotherapy of B cell neoplasms with an anti-B4-blocked ricin: A phase I trial of daily bolus infusion. Blood 79:576, 1992.

24. Appelbaum FR, Matthews DC, Eary JF, et al: Use of radiolabeled anti-Cd33 antibody to augment marrow irradiation prior to marrow transplantation for acute myelogenous leukemia. Transplantation 54:829, 1992.

25. Dillman RO: Monoclonal antibodies for treating cancer. Ann Intern Med 111:592, 1989.

26. Ritz J, Pesando JM, Sallan SE, et al: Serotherapy of acute lymphoblastic leukemia with monoclonal antibody. Blood 58:141, 1981.

27. Dillman RO, Beauregard JC, Halpern SE, et al: Toxicities and side effects associated with intravenous infusions of murine monoclonal antibodies. J Biol Response Mod 5:73, 1986.

28. Nadler LM, Stashenko P, Hardy R, et al: Serotherapy of a patient with a monoclonal antibody directed against a human lymphoma-associated antigen. Cancer Res 40:3147, 1980.

29. Press OW, Appelbaum F, Ledbetter JA, et al: Monoclonal anti-

body 1F5 (anti-CD20) serotherapy of human B-cell lymphomas. Blood 69:584, 1987.

30. Miller RA, Maloney DG, Warnke R, et al: Treatment of a B cell lymphoma with monoclonal anti-idiotype antibody. N Engl J Med 306:517, 1982.
31. Miller R, Oseroff AR, Stratte PT, et al: Monoclonal antibody therapeutic trials in seven patients with T-cell lymphoma. Blood 62:988, 1983.
32. Knox SJ, Levy R, Hodgkinson S, et al: Observations on the effect of chimeric anti-CD4 monoclonal antibody in patients with mycosis fungoides. Blood 77:20, 1991.
33. Tanimoto M, Scheinberg DA, Cordon-Cardo C, et al: Restricted expression of an early myeloid and monocytic cell surface antigen defined by monoclonal M195. Leukemia 3:339, 1989.
34. Shen L, Guyre PM, Anderson CL, et al: Heteroantibody-mediated cytotoxicity: Antibody to the high affinity Fc receptor for IgG mediates cytotoxicity by human monocytes that is enhanced by interferon-g and is not blocked by human IgG1. J Immunol 137:3378, 1986.
35. Dyer MJS, Hale G, Hayhoe FGJ, et al: Effects of CAMPATH-1 antibodies in vivo in patients with lymphoid malignancies: Influence of antibody isotype. Blood 73:1431, 1989.
36. Brown SL, Miller RA, Horning SJ, et al: Treatment of B-cell lymphoma with anti-idiotype antibodies alone and in combination with alpha interferon. Blood 73:651, 1989.
37. Swisher EM, Shawler DL, Collins HA, et al: Expression of shared idiotypes in chronic lymphocytic leukemia and small lymphocytic lymphoma. Blood 77:1977, 1991.
38. Meeker T, Lowder J, Cleary ML, et al: Emergence of idiotype variants during treatment of B cell lymphomas with anti-idiotype antibodies. N Engl J Med 312:1658, 1985.
39. Chatterjee M, Barcos M, Han T, et al: Shared idiotype expression by chronic lymphocytic leukemia and B-cell lymphoma. Blood 76:1825, 1990.
40. Waldman TA, Pastan IH, Gansow OA, et al: The multichain interkeukin-2 receptor: A target for immunotherapy. Ann Intern Med 116:148, 1992.
41. Waldman TA, Goldman CK, Bongiovanni KF, et al: Therapy of patients with human T-cell lymphotrophic virus I-induced adult T-cell leukemia with anti-Tac, a monoclonal antibody to the receptor for interkeukin-2. Blood 72:1805, 1988.
42. Ball ED, Bernier GM, Cornwell GG III, et al: Monoclonal antibodies to myeloid differentiation antigens: In vivo studies of

three patients with acute myeloid leukemia. Blood 62:1203, 1983.

43. Wagner J, Johnson R, Santos G, et al: Systemic monoclonal antibody therapy for eliminating minimal residual leukemia in a rat bone marrow transplant model. Blood 73:614, 1989.
44. Scheinberg DA, Lovett D, Chaitanya R, et al: A phase I trial of monoclonal antibody M195 in acute myelogenous leukemia: Specific bone marrow targeting and internalization of radionuclide. J Clin Oncol 9:478, 1991.
45. Scheinberg DA, Tanimoto M, McKenzie S, et al: Monoclonal antibody M195: A diagnostic marker for acute myelogenous leukemia. Leukemia 3:440, 1989.

Chapter 5

Interleukin-2 as Graft-Versus-Host Disease Prophylaxis

Megan Sykes, M.D.

Despite major advances in immunosuppressive therapy and supportive care, bone marrow transplantation (BMT) has yet to realize its full potential for the treatment of leukemia and other disorders. The major obstacle to further advancement is graft-versus-host disease (GVHD), which can best be prevented by removing T cells from the marrow. However, T-cell depletion has unfortunately been associated with increased rates of engraftment failure[1] and increased relapse rates for several types of leukemia.[2,3] Despite widespread use of cyclosporin A (CsA) and methotrexate for GVHD prophylaxis, significant GVHD is still a major complication of 30% to 40% of human leukocyte antigen (HLA)-matched transplants, and its even greater incidence in the presence of HLA mismatches limits the application of BMT across extensive HLA barriers.[4] Allogeneic BMT, consequently, has not yet realized its full potential for the treatment of leukemia, since most potential recipients unfortunately do not have an HLA-matched sibling donor. Although matched, unrelated donors have made BMT available to an additional fraction of patients, the use of such donors has been associated with a very high incidence of GVHD,[5-7] probably because of the presence of nonserologically detectable HLA mismatches

This work was supported by NIH grants #CA55290, AI31158 and HL49915. Dr. Sykes is supported by an American Cancer Society Junior Faculty Research Award.

From: Spitzer T, Mazumder A: Immunotherapy and Bone Marrow Transplantation. Armonk, NY, Futura Publishing Co., Inc., © 1995.

between members of such pairs, and possibly because of the greater number of minor antigenic disparities that exist between unrelated individuals.

We have recently developed a murine model which appears to preserve the beneficial graft-versus-leukemia (GVL) and engraftment-promoting effects of allogeneic T cells, while inhibiting GVHD across complete major histocompatibility complex (MHC) barriers. Our studies demonstrated that administration of a high dose of interleukin (IL)-2 for 2 1/2 days, beginning on the day of BMT, protects lethally irradiated mice against GVHD mortality in completely MHC- plus multiple minor histocompatibility antigen (miHA)-mismatched murine strain combinations, especially when T-cell-depleted (TCD) host-type bone marrow cells (BMC) (ie, syngeneic marrow; the human counterpart would be autologous or identical twin marrow) were coadministered (Figure 1).[8]

In contrast to the effect of donor marrow T-cell depletion, alloengraftment was not significantly inhibited by IL-2 in the above,[8] or in other more sensitive models evaluating engraftment.[9] Importantly, the engraftment-promoting effect of donor T cells was shown to be preserved in IL-2-treated mice in a sublethal irradiation model in which alloengraftment was T-cell-dependent, as it often is in the clinical situation.[9]

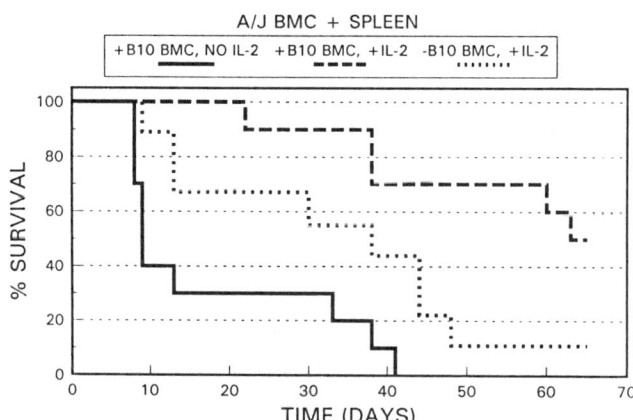

Figure 1. Protective effect of IL-2 plus T-cell-depleted host-type marrow against GVHD in a fully MHC-mismatched strain combination. Survival is shown for lethally irradiated B10 (H-2^b) recipients of allogeneic A/J (H-2^a) BMC and spleen cells plus TCD host-type (B10) BMC (____) with no further treatment, or with 50,000 Units of recombinant human IL-2 twice daily for two days (day 0 to 2) (____). A third group (.........) received similar IL-2 treatment but did not receive TCD host-type BMC with the allogeneic BMC and spleen cells.

Graft-Versus-Leukemia Activities in Interleukin-2-Protected Mice

Since IL-2 had such a potent inhibitory effect on GVHD, we were concerned that, like T-cell depletion, it might also reduce GVL effects of donor T cells. However, in two leukemic models we have studied, no inhibition of the GVL effect of allogeneic T cells was observed in animals receiving IL-2 as GVHD prophylaxis. The first model involved a T-cell leukemia/lymphoma, EL4.[10] In an effort to explain the dissociation of GVHD and GVL in this model, we examined the T-cell subsets involved in producing GVHD and GVL effects. These studies showed that the cluster designation (CD)8+ T-cell subset alone was responsible for the antileukemic effect of donor T cells (Figure 2), and that donor CD4+ T cells played a critical role in inducing

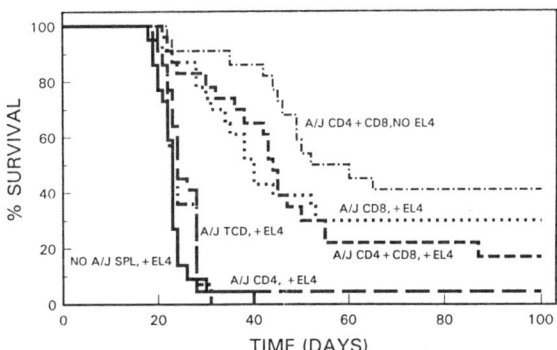

Figure 2. GVL against EL4 leukemia/lymphoma is mediated by CD8+ T cells and not CD4+ T cells in IL-2-treated mice. The combined results of three experiments, all yielding similar results, are shown. All mice were treated with IL-2, 50 000 U twice daily for five doses (day 0 to 2). Lethally irradiated B10 mice received 500 EL4 cells and TCD B10 BMC either without A/J spleen cells (____; N=22) or with A/J BMC and A/J spleen cells treated with: C alone (____; N=23); anti-CD4/C (.........; N=23); anti-CD8/C (_____; N=22); or anti-CD4/anti-CD8/C (__..__; N=14). An additional group (_._._._; N=22) received TCD B10 BMC and A/J BMC, and C-treated A/J spleen cells to control for GVHD mortality. Previous studies have shown that EL4 does not influence GVHD mortality (our unpublished data), so the difference in mortality between recipients of A/J spleen cells with versus without EL4 cells is due to leukemia. An additional control group (not shown; N=10) received TCD syngeneic BMC only, and demonstrated 100% 100-day survival. In some experiments, the leukemic control group (____) also received A/J BMC, but mortality was similar to that of control groups receiving only B10 BMC with EL4, consistent with previous results showing that A/J BMC have no additional GVL effect in this model.[32] Reprinted with permission from the Journal of Immunology 150:197, 1993. Copyright 1993, The Journal of Immunology.

GVHD in this and other fully MHC-mismatched strain combinations.[11,12] IL-2 inhibited only CD4-dependent T-cell activities, such as GVHD, and did not inhibit CD4-independent, CD8-mediated activites such as the GVL effect against EL4.[11] The ability of IL-2 treatment to inhibit the function of donor CD4+ cells and not of CD4-independent CD8+ cells therefore provided an explanation for the dissociation of GVHD and GVL in this model.

However, both murine and human studies suggest that CD4+ cells can also mediate GVL effects against some leukemias.[13,14] We considered the possibility that, since IL-2 inhibits the GVHD-producing activity of CD4+ cells, it might also inhibit CD4-mediated GVL effects. We therefore developed an additional leukemia model involving a promonocytic leukemia called 2B-4-2 (the model is shown in Figure 3). This leukemia is established in vivo prior to irradiation and BMT. Lethal irradiation and syngeneic BMT results in only a few days' prolongation of survival compared to that in nontransplanted mice, and death generally occurs 2 to 4 weeks following BMT. Since this leukemia expresses Class II MHC in addition to Class I

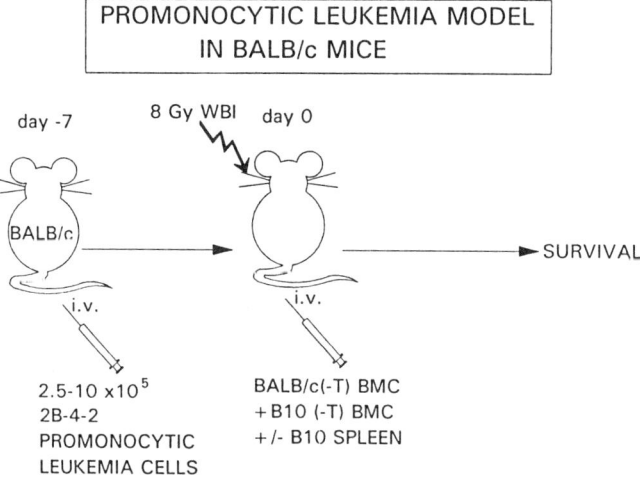

Figure 3. Promonocytic leukemia model. The 2B-4-2 leukemia was derived from pristane-primed BALB/c mice that had received an IV injection of M-MuLV.[33] The cells express both Class I and Class II MHC, as well as Mac-1, and do not express Thy1 or sIgM. BALB/c recipient mice are treated with 2B-4-2 one week prior to irradiation, so that tumor is established in vivo at the time of BMT.

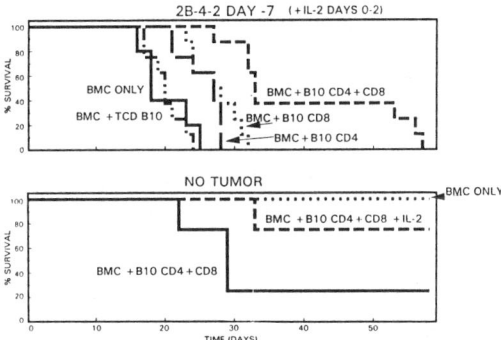

Figure 4. A: BALB/c mice received 2.5×10^5 2B-4-2 cells intravenously on day 7, followed by 8 Gy WBI on day 0, and IV administration of 7×10^6 TCD B10 BMC and 5×10^6 TCD BALB/c BMC alone (___;n=5) or with 12×10^6 B10 spleen cells treated with: C only (____, n=8; inoculum contained 2.19×10^6 CD4+ and 0.89×10^6 CD8+ cells); anti-CD4/C (.........,n=8; inoculum contained 0.007×10^6 CD4+ and 0.85×10^6 CD8+ cells); anti-CD8/C (_____,n=8; inoculum contained 2.0×10^6 CD4+ plus 0.048×10^6 CD8+ cells), or anti-CD4 plus anti-CD8/C (__.._,n=8; inoculum contained a total of 0.043×10^6 CD4+ and CD8+ cells). All mice received IL-2, 5×10^4 Cetus Units i.p. twice daily from day 0 to 2 (5 doses). B: IL-2 protects against GVHD in nonleukemic control mice in the same experiment. Animals received similar inocula as those in the top panel, without receiving tumor. Recipients of BMC only (.........;n=4); BMC plus C-treated B10 spleen cells (___;n=4); BMC plus C-treated B10 spleen cells plus IL-2 (____;n=8). Reprinted with permission from Blood, Vol. 83, 1994.

MHC molecules, we suspected that allogeneic CD4+ cells, in addition to CD8+ T cells, might resist its growth. Indeed, allogeneic, but not syngeneic, T cells of both the CD4+ and CD8+ subsets mediated GVL effects against this leukemia (Figure 4). IL-2 neither enhanced nor inhibited these GVL effects, but did inhibit GVHD. When we compared GVL mediated by allogeneic CD4+ cells in the presence or absence of IL-2 treatment, we found that the magnitude of this CD4-mediated GVL effect was not reduced, even though CD4-mediated GVHD was inhibited in the same mice by IL-2.[15] Thus, using a short course of IL-2 treatment, the GVL- and GVHD-producing effects of a single phenotypic subset of T cells, the CD4-positives, can be dissociated. In addition, CD8-mediated GVL effects against two different leukemias were unaffected by IL-2 treatment. Therefore, treatment with IL-2 dissociated GVHD and GVL effects of alloreactive T cells by at least two different mechanisms.

Studies to Determine Which Types of Histocompatibility Barriers Are Most Amenable to the Protective Effect of Interleukin-2

We have confirmed the ability of IL-2 to inhibit the function of GVHD-promoting CD4+ T cells, and its inability to inhibit the function of CD4-independent, CD8+ cells in several additional strain combinations. In total, 10 different fully MHC-mismatched strain combinations have been evaluated (including 1 P→F1 combination), and IL-2 has been found to inhibit GVHD in 9 of them. CD4+ T cells were found to play a predominant role in producing acute GVHD in all four of four such strain combinations examined.[12] The inability of IL-2 to inhibit CD8-mediated GVHD has been confirmed in several strain combinations, including two that involved isolated Class I MHC disparities (B6→bm1×B6 and B10.AKM→B10.MBR) and one that involved miHA only (B10→C3H.SW).[12]

Thus, the studies described above are consistent with the following generalizations:

1. IL-2 inhibits the GVHD-promoting activity of CD4+ T cells, and not of CD4-independent CD8+ T cells;
2. acute, lethal GVHD in most fully MHC-mismatched strain combinations is largely dependent on the activity of donor CD4+ T cells; and
3. not all CD4 activities are inhibited by IL-2. Importantly, CD4-mediated GVL effects are not inhibited by IL-2.

Failure of Major Histocompatibility Complex Disparities to Increase the Severity of Graft-Versus-Host Disease When CD8+ Cells Are Given Without CD4+ Cells

In view of the ability of CD8+ T cells (given without CD4+ cells) to cause GVHD in mice mismatched at minor histocompatibility or Class I MHC loci alone,[16,17] we have been surprised by their relatively weak capacity to cause acute GVHD in several fully MHC- plus miHA-mismatched strain combinations, which include both minor and Class I MHC disparities.[11,12,18-22] We have directly addressed the question of whether or not adding MHC disparities increases the severity of CD8-mediated GVHD. We took advantage of the existence of congenic and MHC recombinant mouse strains, so that we could evaluate GVHD induced by a single donor strain in recipient strains that all express the same minor histocompatibility differences from the donor, but that do or do not differ at various MHC loci. Thus, it was possible to determine the effect of adding MHC disparities on GVHD mediated by CD8$^+$ cells. These studies showed that adding partial or complete (K, D, both alleles) Class I disparity, or complete Class I plus Class II disparities to minor antigenic disparities resulted in either no difference, or a delay in the onset of GVHD in lethally irradiated recipients of CD4-depleted marrow and spleen cells from a single donor strain (M. Sykes, unpublished data). Therefore, the ability of CD8$^+$ T cells given without CD4$^+$ cells to produce GVHD does not increase as the degree of histoincompatibility increases. The implication of this finding for clinical BMT is that, if marrow were thoroughly CD4-depleted and conventional immunosuppressive pharmacoprophylaxis were used, the incidence of GVHD in HLA-mismatched BMT might be expected to be no greater than that observed in HLA-matched sibling transplantation. However, the alternative to CD4 cell depletion, using IL-2 to diminish CD4-mediated GVHD, has the advantage of preserving GVL effects of this T-cell subset.

Mechanism of Interleukin-2-Induced Inhibition of CD4 Function

A variety of possible mechansims for the anti-GVHD effect of IL-2 have been considered. This protective effect does not appear to depend on donor or host natural killer (NK) cells, lymphokine-activated killer (LAK) cells,[23] or radioresistant CD8$^+$ host T cells (V.S. Abraham and M. Sykes, unpublished data). IL-2 treatment reduces donor T-cell numbers in the first few days following BMT, and increases the percentage of cells expressing the CD3$^+$CD4$^-$CD8$^-$ phenotype.[24] These cells express αβ-T-cell receptor (TCR) and are of both donor and host type (M. Sykes, unpublished data). This phenotype is similar to that on a bone marrow (BM)-derived cell population which has suppressive activity in vitro and can inhibit GVHD.[25,26] We are currently investigating the possibility that these cells might be responsible for the anti-GVHD effect of IL-2.

Additional studies have shown that the protective effect of IL-2 against GVHD requires the presence of IL-2 at the time of donor T-cell contact with host antigen. Pretreatment of hosts with IL-2 before allogeneic BMT does not induce GVHD protection,[27] and pretreatment of donors with IL-2 is also ineffective (M. Sykes, unpublished data). However, IL-2 does inhibit GVHD induced by previously sensitized (to host antigens) donor T cells.[11] The inhibitory effect of IL-2 is not associated with clonal deletion, global anergy or failure of activation of host-reactive cells. Limiting dilution analyses have shown that marked expansion of host-reactive T-helper cells (Th) occurs, to a similar extent, in GVHD control and IL-2-treated mice in the first week post-BMT, and that an extraordinarily high proportion of T cells from both groups are in an activated state (M. Sykes, unpublished data)

The observation that the GVL effect of alloreactive CD4+ cells is completely preserved while their GVHD-promoting activity is diminished by IL-2 treatment suggests that different activities of CD4+ T cells may contribute to each effect. Indeed, CD4+ T cells are not homogeneous in their functions. Two subsets of murine and human CD4+ helper T cells have recently been defined, each of which produces a distinct pattern of cytokines.[28,29] Only Th1 cells produce interferon (IFN)-γ and IL-2, whereas IL-4, IL-5, IL-6 and IL-10 are produced exclusively by cells of the Th2 subset in the mouse. A similar dichotomy has been described for human Th,[29] although IL-10 can be made by both Th1 and Th2 clones of the human.[30] Some cytokines, such as IL-3 and granulocyte macrophage-colony stimulating factor (GM-CSF), are produced by both subsets. Some CD4+ T cells can also mediate cytolytic activity. In an effort to determine which activities of CD4+ cells are inhibited by IL-2 treatment, we have begun to evaluate cytokine production by the expanded and activated host-reactive Th present in GVHD control and IL-2-protected mice. Studies of sera and of in vitro cytokine production indicate that IL-2 treatment inhibits the marked increase in IFN-γ production that is observed in the first 3 to 5 days following BMT in our A/J (H-2^a)→B10 (H-2^b) BMT model, and increases the production of IL-4, a cytokine that is associated with the Th2 CD4 subset. These cytokines are produced predominantly by CD4+ cells on day 4 following BMT, suggesting that IL-2 treatment may change a normally Th1-associated GVH response to a Th2-dominant response (M. Wang, J. Szebeni and M. Sykes, unpublished data). However, we have not detected differences in IL-2 (Th1 cytokine) or IL-10 (Th2 cytokine) production between the two groups. No changes in the production of the pro-inflammatory cytokines IL-1 or tumor necrosis factor (TNF)-α have been observed in IL-2-protected compared to GVHD control mice (M. Wang, J. Szebeni, M. Sykes, unpublished data). Improved understanding of the mechanism by which IL-2 diminishes GVHD should allow the further development of precise manipulations of the graft-versus-host (GVH) response that preserve GVL effects while attenuating GVHD pathophysiology.

Determination of the Minimal Interleukin-2 Dosing Regimen Required for Optimal Graft-Versus-Host Disease Protection

Since the administration of prolonged IL-2 treatments has been associated with significant toxicity in patients, it will be important to administer the lowest possible dose that has maximal prophylactic activity if IL-2 is to be evaluated in man. In the murine model, we have found that three treatments with IL-2, given at approximately 15, 25, and 40 hours post-BMT, provides GVHD protection that is similar to that observed with a more prolonged, five-treatment course. We have also seen that more frequent (three times daily compared to twice daily) administration of the same total IL-2 dose does not result in any further improvement in GVHD protection. CsA does not interfere with the protective effect of IL-2. Therefore, these two modalities could potentially be combined in patients undergoing allogeneic BMT.[34]

Conclusions

Together, our results suggest that IL-2 might provide effective clinical GVHD prophylaxis in donor-host combinations involving Class II MHC disparities, since CD4+ cells recognize this type of alloantigen. This possibility is currently being evaluated in a preclinical porcine Class II-mismatched BMT model, with encouraging preliminary results (T. Sablinski and D.H. Sachs, personal communication, 1994). In addition, CD4+ cells may contribute to GVHD directed against minor disparities. If Class I MHC disparities were also present in a particular donor-host combination, CD8 depletion might be needed to avoid GVHD directed against these antigens. Although chronic GVHD mortality is not eliminated by IL-2 treatment when severe early mortality occurs in control recipients (eg, Figure

1), IL-2 does reduce chronic GVHD mortality and manifestations in some strain combinations in which sufficient GVHD control animals survive the early period to allow comparison at later time points.[8,12] Since fully MHC and multiple minor antigen-mismatched BMT induces the most severe GVHD, determination of the efficacy of IL-2 as GVHD prophylaxis must await preclinical and clinical trials in the setting of various types of histoincompatibility. Clinical trials are underway at the Massachusetts General Hospital to evaluate the toxicities and GVHD prophylactic efficacy of high dose, short course IL-2 treatment following HLA-matched and mismatched donor allotransplantation for refractory hematologic malignancy. These pilot trials should provide the basis for exploring additional anti-GVHD interventions, such as selective T-cell subset depletion or coadministration of autologous regulatory cell populations, particularly for patients receiving transplants from extensively mismatched donors.

The major attractions of IL-2 treatment compared to the use of BM T-cell depletion for GVHD prophylaxis include:

1. the preserved alloengraftment-promoting effects of allogeneic T cells in IL-2-treated recipients; and
2. the preserved GVL effect of allogeneic T cells in IL-2-treated recipients.

Our studies demonstrate clearly that GVHD-promoting effects can be dissociated from GVL effects of alloreactive donor T cells. If GVHD could be avoided while BMT was performed across broad HLA disparities, then much more potent GVL effects than those observed for HLA-matched transplants might be expected, as we have observed in the murine model.[31]

Acknowledgments: I wish to thank Drs. Lorri A. Lee and Thomas R. Spitzer for critical review of the manuscript.

References

1. Martin PJ, Hansen JA, Torok-Storb B, et al: Graft failure in patients receiving T cell-depleted HLA-identical allogeneic marrow transplants. Bone Marrow Transplant 3:445-456, 1988.
2. Poynton CH: T cell depletion in bone marrow transplantation. Bone Marrow Transplant 3:265-279, 1988.
3. Butturini A, Gale RP: T cell depletion in bone marrow transplantation for leukemia: Current results and future directions. Bone Marrow Transplant 3:265-279, 1988.

4. Clift RA, Storb R: Histoincompatible bone marrow transplants in humans. Annu Rev Immunol 5:43-64, 1987.

5. Ash RC, Horowitz MM, Gale RP, et al: Bone marrow transplantation from related donors other than HLA-identical siblings: Effect of T cell depletion. Bone Marrow Transplant 7:443-452, 1991.

6. McGlave P, Bartsch G, Anasetti C, et al: Unrelated donor marrow transplantation therapy for chronic myelogenous leukemia: Initial experience of the national marrow donor program. Blood 81:543-550, 1993.

7. Kernan NA, Bartsch G, Ash RC, et al: Analysis of 462 transplantations from unrelated donors facilitated by the national marrow donor program. N Engl J Med 328:593-602, 1993.

8. Sykes M, Romick ML, Hoyles KA, et al: In vivo administration of interleukin 2 plus T cell-depleted syngeneic marrow prevents graft-versus-host disease mortality and permits alloengraftment. J Exp Med 171:645-658, 1990.

9. Sykes M, Pearson DA: Alloengraftment in IL-2-treated mice. Bone Marrow Transplant 10:157-163, 1992.

10. Sykes M, Romick ML, Sachs DH: Interleukin 2 prevents graft-vs-host disease while preserving the graft-vs-leukemia effect of allogeneic T cells. Proc Natl Acad Sci U S A 87:5633-5637, 1990.

11. Sykes M, Abraham VS, Harty MW, et al: IL-2 reduces graft-vs-host disease and preserves a graft-vs-leukemia effect by selectively inhibiting CD4+ T cell activity. J Immunol 150:197- 205, 1993.

12. Sykes M, Harty MW, Pearson DA: Strain dependence of IL-2-induced GVHD protection: Evidence that IL-2 inhibits selected CD4 functions. J Immunother 15:11-21, 1994.

13. Champlin R, Ho W, Gajewski J, et al: Selective depletion of CD8+ T lymphocytes for prevention of graft-versus-host disease after allogeneic bone marrow transplantation. Blood 76:418-423, 1990.

14. Truitt RL, Atasoylu AA: Contribution of CD4+ and CD8+ T cells to graft-versus-host disease and graft-versus-leukemia reactivity after transplantation of MHC-compatible bone marrow. Bone Marrow Transplant 8:51-58, 1991.

15. Sykes M, Harty MW, Szot GL, et al: IL-2 inhibits graft-versus-host-disease-promoting activity of CD4+ cells while preserving CD4- and CD8-mediated graft-vs-leukemia effects. Blood 83:-2560-2569, 1994.

16. Sprent J, Schaefer M, Gao E, et al: Role of T cell subsets in lethal graft-versus host disease (GVHD) directed to class I versus class II H-2 differences. I. L3T4+ cells can either augment or retard

GVHD elicited by Lyt-2+ cells in ClassI-different hosts. J Exp Med 167:556-569, 1988.

17. Korngold R, Sprent J: Variable capacity of L3T4+ T cells to cause lethal graft-versus-host disease across minor histocompatibility barriers in mice. J Exp Med 165:1552-1564, 1987.

18. Pietryga D, Blazar BR, Soderling CB, et al: The effect of T subset depletion on the incidence of lethal graft-versus-host disease in a murine major-histocompatibility-complex-mismatched transplantation system. Transplantation 43:442-445, 1987.

19. Korngold R, Sprent J: Surface markers of T cells causing lethal graft-vs-host disease to class I vs class II H-2 differences. J Immunol 135:3004-3010, 1985.

20. Vallera DA, Soderling CCB, Kersey JH: Bone marrow transplantation across major histocompatibility barriers in mice. III. Treatment of donor grafts with monoclonal antibodies directed against Lyt determinants. J Immunol 128:871-876,1982.

21. Uenaka A, Mieno M, Kuribayashi K, et al: Effector cells of lethal graft-versus-host disease (GVHD) in nude mice. Transplant Proc 21:3031-3032, 1989.

22. Thiele DL, Charley MR, Calomeni JA, et al: Lethal graft-vs-host disease across major histocompatibility barriers: Requirement for leucyl-leucine methyl ester sensitive cytotoxic T cells. J Immunol 138:51-57, 1987.

23. Sykes M, Abraham VS: Mechanism of IL-2-mediated protection against GVHD in mice. II. Protection occurs independently of NK/LAK cells. Transplantation 53:1063-1070, 1992.

24. Abraham VS, Sachs DH, Sykes M: The mechanism of protection from GVHD mortality by IL-2. III. Early reductions in donor T cell subsets and expansion of a CD3+CD4-CD8- cell population. J Immunol 148:3746-3752, 1992.

25. Sykes M, Hoyles KA, Romick ML, et al: In vitro and in vivo analysis of bone marrow derived CD3+, CD4-, CD8-, NK1.1+ cell lines. Cell Immunol 129:478-493, 1990.

26. Palathumpat V, Dejbakhsh-Jones S, Holm B, et al: Different subsets of T cells in the adult mouse bone marrow and spleen induce or suppress acute graft-versus-host disease. J Immunol 149:808-817, 1992.

27. Abraham VS, Sykes M: Mechanism of the anti-GVHD effect of IL-2. I. Protective host-type cell populations are not induced by IL-2 treatment alone. Bone Marrow Transplant 7(Supp 1):29-32, 1991.

28. Mossman TR, Coffman RL: Th1 and Th2 cells: Different patterns of lymphokine secretion lead to different functional properties. Annu Rev Immunol 7:145-154, 1989.

29. Romagnani S: Human Th1 and Th2 subsets: Doubt no more. Immunol Today 12:256-257, 1991.
30. Yssel H, de Waal Malefyt R, Roncarolo MG, et al: IL-10 is produced by subsets of human CD4+ T cell clones and peripheral blood T cells. J Immunol 149:2378-2384, 1992.
31. Sykes M, Sachs DH: Genetic analysis of the anti-leukemic effect of mixed allogeneic bone marrow transplantation. Transplant Proc 21:3022-3024, 1989.
32. Sykes M, Bukhari Z, Sachs DH: Graft-versus-leukemia effect using mixed allogeneic bone marrow transplantation. Bone Marrow Transplant 4:465-474, 1989.
33. Wolff L, Mushinski JF, Shen-Ong GLC, et al: A chronic inflammatory response. Its role in supporting the development of c-myb and c-myc related promonocytic and monocytic tumors in BALB/c mice. J Immunol 141:681-689, 1988.
34. Sykes M: IL-2-induced GVHD protection is not inhibited by cyclosporin A and is maximal when IL-2 is given over a 25-hour period beginning on the day following bone marrow transplantation. Bone Marrow Transplant 1994. In press.

Chapter 6

Interleukin-2 as Consolidative Immunotherapy After Clinical Autologous Bone Marrow Transplantation

Alexander Fefer, M.D., Mark C. Benyunes, M.D.

Background and Rationale for Interleukin-2 Therapy as an Adjunct to Autologous Bone Marrow Transplantation

The success of autologous bone marrow transplantation (BMT) for patients with hematologic malignancies is limited largely by a high incidence of posttransplant relapses. This has been attributed to residual malignant cells which have survived the preparative regimens for autologous BMT, and/or tumor cells which may have been infused with the marrow. Attempts to decrease the relapse rate by adding more chemotherapy or radiation to the conditioning regimens

This work was supported in part by Grants PO1 CA-47748, CA-18029, CA-15704, and T32 CA-09515, awarded by the National Cancer Institute, the Department of Health and Human Services, the Jose Carreras International Leukemia Foundation and the Jennie Zoline Foundation.

for autologous BMT have been hampered by the cross-resistance of the tumor to the various agents, and by their shared cumulative toxicities. Moreover, although elegant recent studies using genetic markers have demonstrated the presence of leukemic cells originating in the infused marrow in two patients,[1] the degree to which such contamination is responsible for, or contributes to, the ultimate clinical relapses in any given patient or in a population of patients who have undergone autologous BMT and relapsed is not known. Nevertheless, a variety of approaches to purging autologous marrow of tumor cells prior to transplantation have been almost routinely used by most investigators. However, no conclusive evidence of a long-term benefit of such purging has been provided, largely because no Phase III randomized trial of purged versus nonpurged marrow has been reported.

It is postulated that posttransplant immunotherapy with Interleukin (IL)-2, with or without the transfer of lymphocytes possessing specific or nonspecific antitumor reactivities, might decrease the relapse rate following autologous BMT by eradicating residual tumor cells which survived the preparative regimen, as well as any clonogenic malignant cells which contaminated the infused marrow. The basis for this hypothesis is described below.

1. Human leukemia cells, including acute myeloid leukemia (AML), acute lymphoblastic leukemia (ALL), and chronic myeloid leukemia (CML), as well as lymphoma and myeloma cells, can be lysed by lymphokine-activated killer (LAK) cells in vitro.[2-4] Susceptibility to such lysis is not cell-cycle specific and is maintained in cell lines which demonstrate pleiotropic drug-resistance markers.[5,6] In addition to being directly lytic, LAK cells or activated-natural killer (A-NK) cells also inhibit malignant colony proliferation in assays of clonogenic tumor growth.[7,8]

2. Thus, since tumor cell lines resistant to chemotherapeutic agents remain susceptible to LAK-mediated lysis in vitro,[5] IL-2-based immunotherapy is potentially noncross-resistant with chemo-radiotherapy.

3. Some patients with advanced hematologic malignancies including malignant lymphoma (ML)[9-12] and AML[13-16] refractory to conventional therapy or even to autologous BMT, have responded to IL-2 ± LAK cells with partial or, occasionally, complete clinical responses.[17]

4. Immunotherapy should theoretically be more effective in a setting of minimal residual disease—such as that which is attained by the conditioning regimens used for autologous BMT.

5. IL-2 therapy after autologous BMT should theoretically be able to eradicate whatever clonogenic malignant cells might be present in the infused marrow—a form of purging in vivo which should obviate the need for purging the marrow of tumor cells in vitro.

6. Finally, IL-2 therapy after autologous BMT induces clinical and histopathological cutaneous graft-versus-host disease (GVHD) in most patients,[18] and might induce or amplify a graft-versus-leukemia (GVL) effect.[19]

Although the most cogent circumstantial clinical evidence for the existence of a GVL effect has been derived in the setting of allogeneic BMT, namely that relapse rates are lower in recipients of allogeneic BMT who develop GVHD than in those without GVHD or in recipients of syngeneic or T-depleted allogeneic marrow,[19] a GVL effect could theoretically also exist after autologous BMT, but may not be readily demonstrable because of the lack of appropriate negative controls. GVL after autologous BMT might be mediated by lymphocytes which, unlike cells in syngeneic marrow recipients, have been exposed to and "immunized" against putative tumor-associated antigens pretransplant, and which, when reinfused with the autologous marrow, might eradicate the smaller numbers of tumor cells remaining after cytoreductive therapy. Effector cells which might mediate a GVL effect after autologous BMT may include:

1. cytotoxic T-lymphocytes (CTL) specific for antigens expressed only or preferentially by malignant cells;

2. cytolytic T cells or non-T cells that mediate their antitumor effect by a major histocompatibility complex (MHC)-unrestricted mechanism; and/or

3. cells which mediate their antitumor effects via secretion of secondary cytokines such as tumor necrosis factor (TNF)-α, interferon (IFN)-γ, granulocyte macrophage-colony stimulating factor (GM-CSF) and others.

IL-2 can stimulate the proliferation and function of all of the above mentioned effector cells.

This chapter will briefly summarize the results of clinical trials of IL-2± lymphocytes for heavily pretreated malignant lymphoma and acute leukemia patients not undergoing autologous BMT, and the results of the clinical trials of IL-2± lymphocytes after autologous BMT for hematologic malignancies by our group as well as others. These results are sufficiently encouraging to justify launching prospectively randomized Phase III trials of IL-2 versus no IL-2 after autologous BMT for hematologic malignancies at high- risk for relapse. Finally, future research in the directions of using tumor-specific T cells in the context of autologous BMT and IL-2 or other lymphokines will also be covered.

Interleukin-2± Lymphokine Activated Killer Cells as Therapy for Hematologic Malignancies in Humans[17]

Hematologic malignancies are among the most sensitive to chemotherapy and/or radiation. A state of minimal residual disease can, therefore, readily be induced by conventional therapy, as well as by the more aggressive chemo-radiotherapy preparative regimens used for autologous BMT. Therefore, a variety of IL-2 regimens ± LAK cells have been employed to treat an extremely heterogeneous group of patients with hematologic malignancies, with encouraging preliminary results.

Clinical Trials of Interleukin-2 for Malignant Lymphoma

Several Phase I/II trials have included or have been restricted to patients with ML. These patients have generally been heavily pretreated with chemotherapy and/or radiation and some had already relapsed after autologous BMT. This additional exposure to chemotherapy/radiotherapy could influence both the toxicity of and the tumor responses to IL-2 therapy. For example, such patients may be more susceptible to IL-2-induced capillary leak syndrome (CLS) and thrombocytopenia; the latter might be exacerbated by the frequent lymphomatous involvement of the marrow. Moreover, heavily pretreated patients may be less able to respond immunologically to IL-2, with a resultant decrease in the probability of tumor eradication. Nevertheless, Phase I/II trials of IL-2 have initially involved patients with advanced, chemotherapy-resistant ML with a view to subsequent trials in the more favorable situation of minimal residual disease.

The lymphoma patients treated have been heterogeneous with respect to histologic grade, stage, prior therapy, disease sites, and amount of disease at the start of IL-2 therapy. The IL-2 regimens also varied in terms of source, dose, route and schedule of administration. Some of the trials also included exogenously-generated LAK cells. Comparative studies have not been performed to identify the optimal IL-2 regimen or assess the therapeutic contribution, if any, of LAK cells.

The eight trials reported to date include a total of 109 patients, all in relapse, who were treated with some regimen of IL-2 alone (70 patients) or IL-2/LAK cells (39 patients).[11,12,20-24] The IL-2 dose was most often high enough to require hospitalization and, occasionally, intensive care unit management. Overall, of the 109 available patients treated, 7 exhibited a complete response (CR); 15, a partial response (PR), for an overall response rate of 20%.

Responses were noted in lymph nodes, bone marrow (BM), peripheral blood, spleen, liver and skin. The CRs lasted 2 to 23+ months and PRs lasted 1 to 36+ months. The histologic grade of the lymphoma was reported for only 79 of the 109 patients treated. Of 40 patients with high-grade non-Hodgkin's lymphoma (NHL) treated with IL-2± LAK cells, 3 exhibited a CR; 4, a PR, for an overall response rate of 18%. Of 39 patients with low-grade NHL, 3 exhibited a CR; 9, a PR, for an overall response rate of 31%.

Interestingly, two of three CRs and one of three PRs reported in the high-grade NHL occurred in patients whose tumors expressed "T-cell" phenotype.[21] Moreover, of four patients treated with IL-2 for refractory heavily pretreated mycosis fungoides, two exhibited a CR; two, a PR. All tumors expressed either the low-affinity IL-2 receptor cluster designation (CD)25, or CD4.[21] Thus, IL-2 therapy can induce significant clinical regressions of T-cell lymphomas in some patients.

Five reports of clinical trials of IL-2± LAK cells have included 28 patients with Hodgkin's disease (HD),[20-23,25] all extensively pretreated, and 8 who had relapsed after autologous BMT. One PR, and for 11 months, 3 brief PRs (all ≤3 months) were observed.

Clearly, some regimens of IL-2, with or without LAK cells, can induce a PR or even a CR in some patients with ML. However, the therapies and the patients have been too heterogeneous to permit any conclusions regarding the optimal IL-2 regimens, the contribution of LAK cells, if any, or the identification of any subset of patients who are more or less likely to benefit from IL-2 therapy.

Clinical Trials of Interleukin-2 for Acute Leukemia[26]

IL-2 therapy has also been reported to have activity in some patients with acute leukemia who had relapsed after conventional chemotherapy or after autologous BMT. High-dose IL-2 administered by continuous intravenous infusion (CIV) to treat such AML patients yielded different results, depending on the tumor load at the time that IL-2 therapy was initiated. Among the seven patients who began IL-2 therapy with ≥30% blasts in the marrow, none responded,[13-15] whereas four complete responses were induced among five patients with AML in relapse who had "limited disease" (defined as 8% to 15% blasts in the marrow) at the time IL-2 therapy was begun. One of the four responding patients had relapsed after chemotherapy and two autologous marrow transplants, and remains in CR over 48 months after starting IL-2 therapy.

High dose IL-2 by CIV[16] was administered to 10 heavily pretreated patients with AML who had ≥30% blasts in their marrow at the time IL-2 therapy was begun. CR was induced in the patients, but for only 3 to 4 months.

In summary, various regimens of IL-2, with or without LAK cells, have induced tumor responses in some patients with advanced ML or AML in relapse. Unfortunately, most responses are partial and/or of relatively short duration. Nevertheless, in such a poor risk group of patients, the responses must be considered significant and warrant further investigation in more favorable clinical settings, most obviously in patients with minimal residual disease.

NK and LAK precursor activity has been shown to be present in the blood of leukemia patients who are in remission, but not in the blood of patients in relapse.[2,27,28] This suggests that active disease or high tumor burden may suppress NK or LAK function, or that decreased NK/LAK function may predispose to relapse.

Clinical Trials of Interleukin-2 ± Lymphokine-Activated Killer Cells After Autologous Bone Marrow Transplantation for Hematologic Malignancy

The optimal time for initiating IL-2 therapy after autologous BMT is not known, nor has the optimal dose and regimen been identified. Since relapses most often occur within a few months after autologous BMT,[29-33] IL-2± LAK cell therapy as consolidative immunotherapy would have to be administered early, before the relapses are likely to occur. IL-2-responsive LAK precursor cells, defined as lymphocytes able to lyse Daudi tumor targets in vitro after being incubated in vitro with IL-2, have been detected in the peripheral circulation as early as 2 weeks after autologous BMT.[34-38] Cells with spontaneous LAK effector activity, defined as the ability of lymphocytes to lyse Daudi in vitro without exposure to IL-2 in vitro, can be shown to circulate in the blood of patients within 3 to 6 weeks after autologous BMT.[37,38] Patients thus have the capacity to respond immunologically to IL-2 during this early posttransplant period. However, patients may be more susceptible to IL-2-associated toxicities soon after undergoing high-dose chemo-radiotherapy and autologous BMT. The possibility of myelosuppression by IL-2 was of particular concern, since IL-2-induced anemia and thrombocytopenia had been reported.[39]

Trials of Interleukin-2 after Autologous Bone Marrow Transplantation for Hematologic Malignancies

Several Phase I trials of IL-2 have been performed to determine the toxicity and immunomodulatory effects of IL-2 administered at various times early after autologous BMT. These studies involved different sources, schedules, and regimens of IL-2[34-36]

Severe toxicity was reported in two patients who received high-dose IL-2 (Glaxo Pharmaceuticals; Research Triangle Park, N.C.) 48 hours after autologous BMT for AML, whereas a lower dose of IL-2 administered at a later time by a different route was less toxic.[35] Similarly, Weisdorf et al., reported serious nonhematologic toxicity when Roche IL-2 (Roche Laboratories; Nutley, N.J.) was administered at doses between 0.5 to 2.0×10^6 U/m^2 per day 4 days per week beginning on day 1 after autologous BMT for ALL.[40] In another study, IL-2 (Cetus Corporation; Emeryville, CA) administered by CIV infusion at 3×10^6 U/m^2 per day beginning 2 to 3 months after autologous BMT did not induce significant hematologic toxicity and all nonhematologic toxicity was manageable and reversible.[41] Low doses of IL-2 may be well-tolerated for a long time, even if the infusions are begun very early after autologous BMT. Thus, IL-2 was well-tolerated by seven patients who received IL-2 (Roche) at a dose of 2×10^5 U/m^2 per day beginning 6 to 14 weeks after autologous BMT, for up to 3 months.[42]

IL-2 administered after autologous BMT has induced significant immunomodulatory effects. These include an increase in the percentage of peripheral blood lymphocytes (PBL) expressing the NK/LAK associated surface markers CD16 and CD56, and a concurrent increase in the circulating NK and LAK effector activity.[34,35,42] Similar changes have been seen in the peripheral blood and BM of patients given IL-2 for AML and ALL.[43] In Weisdorf's trial of IL-2 begun immediately after autologous BMT, no enhancement in the recovery of cells with the NK phenotype or in circulating NK activity was detected. However, in many patients toxicity limited the ability to deliver the planned doses of IL-2.

IL-2 administered in high doses is toxic. The frequent toxicities include fever, gastrointestinal symptoms, skin rash, mild hepatic dysfunction, thrombocytopenia, and a CLS characterized by hypotension, fluid retention, oliguria with azotemia, and respiratory distress. Less common toxicities include bacterial infections, neurological complications such as confusion and seizures, arrhythmias and cardiac ischemia.[44-46]

The major hemopoietic toxicity of IL-2 after autologous BMT has been thrombocytopenia of variable severity and of short duration. IL-2 therapy has had no measurable or permanent deleterious effect on the marrow graft. In fact, most patients treated with IL-2 after autologous BMT exhibited lymphocytosis, eosinophilia and neutrophilia. In vitro studies suggest that these phenomena are due to the release of cytokines such as IL-3, GM-CSF and IL-5 from activated lympyhocytes.[34,47-49] Heslop demonstrated that this is due both to increased protein synthesis of cytokines, as well as increased transcription of mRNA in lymphocytes exposed to IL-2 in vivo.[48]

In an effort to develop a regimen of IL-2 plus autologous LAK cells for eventual testing as consolidative immunotherapy early after autologous BMT, a Phase Ib trial of IL-2 administered early after autologous BMT for hematologic malignancies was performed in Seattle, so as to determine its maximal tolerated dose (MTD) and its immunomodulatory effects.[50] The IL-2 regimen was based on prior experience in treating patients with renal cell carcinoma,[51] and with a view to adding LAK cells to the regimen once the MTD of IL-2 was identified. IL-2 (Roche) was administered by CIV infusion to 16 patients beginning 14 to 91 (median: 33) days after autologous BMT. The patients were heterogeneous in terms of diagnosis, stage of disease, and pretransplant conditioning regimens. All had recovered from acute autologous BMT-associated toxicities, and had evidence of marrow engraftment. Eligibility requirements included a neutrophil count >500/mL, platelets >20 000/mL with or without transfusion support, adequate renal and hepatic function, and absence of infection off antibiotics. Patients were sequentially assigned to escalating IL-2 "induction" doses of 0.3 to 4.5×10^6 Roche U/m^2 per day on days 1 to 5 of the IL-2 protocol, and a nonescalating low IL-2 "maintenance" dose of 0.3×10^6 U/m^2 per day on days 12 to 21. Reversible hypotension and thrombocytopenia were the dose-limiting side effects, and the maximum tolerated "induction" dose of IL-2 was 3.0×10^6 Roche U/m^2 per day. The IL-2 regimen induced a marked

"rebound" lymphocytosis and a significant increase in cells expressing CD16 and CD56, with a concomitant increase in circulating LAK
effector and LAK precursor activity. Similar toxicities and immunomodulatory effects have been reported by others.[35,36,40] Thus,
an IL-2 regimen was identified, which could be tolerated early after
autologous BMT, and could induce a number of dose-related immunomodulatory effects.

Feasibility Trial of Interleukin-2/Autologous Lymphokine-Activated Killer Cells After Autologous Bone Marrow Transplantation for Malignant Lymphoma and Acute Myeloid Leukemia

On the assumption, derived from studies in murine models, that
ex vivo-generated LAK cells might contribute to the potential antitumor efficacy of consolidative IL-2 immunotherapy after autologous
BMT, a Phase I/II trial of IL-2/autologous LAK cells was initiated in
patients who had undergone autologous BMT for advanced hematologic malignancies, in order to determine the feasibility of generating and administering LAK cells in large numbers with IL-2 early
after autologous BMT.

Patients who recovered from autologous BMT and met the eligibility criteria for IL-2, received IL-2 at the MTD of 3×10^6 Roche
U/m^2 per day by CIV on days 1 to 5 of the IL-2 protocol, and underwent leukapheresis daily on days 7 to 9. The cells obtained were incubated with IL-2 1000 U/mL for 5 days, and were infused daily on
days 12 to 14. The low-maintenance dose of IL-2 was administered
on days 12 to 21.

Sixteen patients with ML and five with AML were treated with
autologous BMT followed by IL-2 and autologous LAK cells.[52] The
toxicity of IL-2/LAK therapy was comparable to that of IL-2 alone.
However, leukapheresis was associated with marked exacerbation
of thrombocytopenia. This was most severe in the AML patients, in
whom platelet counts decreased to $<10\,000$/mm^3 for 1 to 12 (median:
5) days despite maximal transfusion support.[53] The severity of the
thrombocytopenia in the AML patients was unacceptable, and LAK
cell generation and infusion was, therefore, discontinued.

A median total of 1.4×10^{11} cells were infused per patient. Phe-
notypically, the cells infused were predominantly CD3$^+$, CD8$^+$ and
CD56$^+$, and were highly lytic to Daudi cells. LAK cell infusions were
generally well-tolerated, with only transient fever, rigors, and dys-
pnea which rapidly reversed. The immunological changes observed

with IL-2/LAK therapy were comparable to those previously reported with IL-2 alone.[54]

Clinical Follow-up of 16 Patients Treated with Autologous Bone Marrow Transplantation and Interleukin-2/Lymphokine-Activated Killer for Malignant Lymphoma[52]

Although the ML patients treated were heterogeneous in regards to diagnosis (12 NHL, 4 HD), stage at autologous BMT (7 in first relapse, and 9 in second relapse or later), and conditioning regimen (4 with chemotherapy alone and 12 with chemotherapy and total body irradiation [TBI]), all were considered at high risk for posttransplant relapse. Prior to reinfusion, the marrow from all patients with NHL was purged with monoclonal anti-B-cell antibodies.

The patients began receiving IL-2 a median of 31 days after autologous BMT. One patient died of infection while in CR 14 months after autologous BMT. Seven patients relapsed 5 to 19 (median: 8) months after autologous BMT, while 8 patients remain in continuous CR at 15+ to 31+ (median: 20+) months. Despite the heterogeneity of the patients, these results are encouraging given that, historically, such patients at our institution have had a 60% to 80% probability of early relapse (median: 3 to 4 months).[29]

Based on these clinical results, a prospectively randomized Phase III trial will soon be launched, in which patients with NHL at high risk for relapse will undergo autologous transplantation after a uniform conditioning regimen consisting of cytoxan, VP-16, and TBI. Once they meet the eligibility criteria, they will be randomized to treatment with IL-2 or to observation in order to determine whether consolidative immunotherapy with IL-2 will reduce the relapse rate and increase the probability of disease-free survival. Since autologous peripheral blood stem cell transplantation (PBSCT) is increasingly being used instead of autologous BMT and appears to be associated with accelerated engraftment,[55] the protocol will involve PBSCT instead of autologous BMT. The use of PBSCT is further justified by the findings that there is a rapid reconstitution of CD56+ cells and cells expressing P75, the intermediate affinity IL-2 receptor, as early as 15 days after PBSCT and that this is associated with IL-2-inducible LAK activity.[56] Finally, since Roche IL-2 is no longer available, the IL-2 to be used in the Phase III trial will be an equivalent regimen of Cetus IL-2, as recently identified via a Phase I clinical trial in patients who have undergone autologous BMT.

Clinical Follow-up of Patients Treated with Autologous Bone Marrow Transplantation/Interleukin-2 or Interleukin-2/Lymphokine-Activated Killer for Acute Myeloid Leukemia[52]

Cumulatively, 14 patients received IL-2 or IL-2/LAK cells after autologous BMT for AML in first relapse or at a later stage. The clinical characteristics of the eight AML patients on the Phase I trial of IL-2 alone after autologous BMT have been described.[57] Five patients with AML in first relapse or second CR received IL-2 and autologous LAK cells after autologous BMT. A sixth patient, scheduled to receive IL-2/LAK, developed sepsis during induction IL-2 and, despite the discontinuation of IL-2, developed multi-organ failure and died. The 14 patients underwent autologous BMT in first relapse (9 patients), second CR (3 patients) or second relapse (2 patients), after being conditioned with busulfan (BU), cyclophosphamide (CY) and TBI (11 patients) or BU/CY alone (3 patients). The marrow was purged with 4-HC in 6 patients and not purged in 8 patients. The median duration of their first CR was 12 months.

The median time from autologous BMT to initiation of IL-2 therapy was 51 days (21 to 91). Three patients relapsed at 4, 5, and 10 months, while 10 remain in CR 15+ to 50+ (median: 36+) months after autologous BMT. Four years after autologous BMT, the actuarial risk of relapse for this group of 14 patients is 23% (confidence interval (CI): 12% to 34%) and the probability of disease-free survival is 71% (CI: 59% to 83%).

A historical control group was generated, which consisted of all patients with AML in first relapse or beyond, who underwent autologous BMT at our institution during the same time period with the same preparative and purging regimens, who met the eligibility criteria for IL-2 therapy but did not receive IL-2 either because they refused, or because of financial problems, or because IL-2 was temporarily unavailable to them. No patient who was eligible for IL-2 therapy was excluded from the control group.

Fifteen such historical controls were thus identified. They did not differ significantly from the 14 patients who received IL-2/LAK cells with respect to age, FAB class, number of cycles of induction and consolidation chemotherapy, duration of first CR, use of 4-HC-treated marrow, type of preparative regimen, or time to engraftment. Two of the 15 control patients died of infection at 6 and 11 months, 9 relapsed within a median of 4 months, while 4 remain in CR 17+ to 46+ (median: 26+) months after autologous BMT.

Despite the small number of patients involved, the results of IL-2± LAK therapy after autologous BMT for AML in first relapse or beyond are encouraging; they are better than would be expected from previous reports,[33,58-60] and from our own historical controls.[30] The results also compare favorably with those reported after allogeneic BMT for AML beyond first CR.[61]

The data provide a basis for a Phase III trial, which is about to be initiated through the Southwest Oncology Group as an Intergroup trial in which patients with AML in first relapse or second CR will undergo autologous BMT after being conditioned with BU/CY and who, once they meet the eligibility criteria, will be randomized to receive IL-2, or to observation. The goal will be to determine whether this approach will reduce the relapse rate and, ultimately, improve the disease-free survival. The new regimen involving the equivalent doses of Cetus IL-2 will be employed.

Future Directions

Future laboratory and clinical studies will be directed at inducing or amplifying a graft-versus-tumor (GVT) effect by involving additional lymphokines. Examples include IL-7, which induces LAK activity in lymphocytes from patients who have undergone autologous BMT[62] and IL-12, which has been reported to enhance cytolytic function of lymphocytes from patients after allogeneic BMT.[63]

Future studies are also likely to involve the use of lymphocytes rendered by modern molecular immunological techniques exquisitely specific and reactive to the malignant cells. T cells directed against antigens expressed uniquely by leukemia or lymphoma cells might be therapeutically as effective in this setting of autologous BMT, as T cells directed against minor histocompatibility antigens (miHA) are in the setting of allogeneic BMT, but without the anti-host toxicity. Extensive studies in animal models have shown that T cells specifically immune to malignant cells can cure advanced malignancy, and IL-2 will augment such efficacy[64] Attempts to apply similar T-cell therapy to humans have been hampered largely by lack of identifiable specific immunogens and targets. This problem is being overcome as the molecular structures recognized by T cells are being identified.

The concept that proteins expressed by an altered cancer-related gene, such as a proto-oncogene, are potential T-cell targets is just beginning to be evaluated.[65-76] T cells do not recognize intact proteins, but rather short peptide fragments (8 to 12 amino acids in length) that have been derived from intact protein processed intracellularly, and presented in the cleft of MHC molecules. Thus, the appropriateness of any particular proto-oncogene product to serve as a T-cell target will depend upon:

1. whether the altered segment of protein has the proper molecular configuration or "motif" to bind in the cleft of Class I or Class II MHC molecules;
2. whether the resultant peptide/MHC molecule complex is present at the cell surface of the target cell or antigen-presenting cell in a concentration high enough to stimulate the specific T-cell receptor (TCR); and
3. whether the peptide/MHC molecule complex is within the TCR repertoire of the particular nominated individuals.

Recent studies have shown that cancer-related proteins of each category can be recognized by T cells and can potentially serve as targets for T-cell attack.[65-76]

Several potentially relevant T-cell targets might be considered in the near future. For example, T cells might be generated which are specifically reactive to the idiotype of a particular B-cell lymphoma to be treated. Moreover, T-cell recognition of transforming proteins encoded by mutated *ras* proto-oncogene has already been reported,[66] as has T-cell immunity to the joining region of small p210bcr-abl protein.[67] Whether the joining region segment of bcr-abl protein, which appears to be leukemia-specific, is an appropriate target for T-cell therapy is not yet known, and is under intense investigation. In addition, it is not known whether such an attack would be optimal when generated by Class I MHC-restricted CD8+ T cells or Class II MHC-restricted CD4+ T cells. Should any of the types of tumor-specific antigens being investigated be capable of stimulating the generation of specific T cells, such cells could be identified, expanded, cloned, and eventually infused for therapeutic purposes, similar to the way CD8+ T-cell clones specific for cytomegalovirus (CMV) have been generated, expanded, and infused into marrow recipients.[77] Based on animal data, any specific T-cell therapy approach is more likely to be attempted against minimal residual disease such as that which exists after BMT. Progress in molecular immunology and gene transfer technology suggests that eventually such approaches, which rely more on tumor specificity, may be induced and used preferentially in autologous BMT, so that BMT approaches will be designed to rely less on the noxious and nonspecific effects of chemo-radiotherapy, and more on specific antitumor lymphocytes and lymphokines.

References

1. Brenner M, Rill D, Moen R, et al: Gene-marking to trace origin of relapse after autologous bone-marrow transplantation. Lancet 341:85-86, 1993.
2. Adler A, Chervenick P, Whiteside T, et al: Interleukin-2 induction of lymphokine-activated killer (LAK) activity in the peripheral blood and bone marrow of acute leukemia patients. I. Feasibility of LAK generation in adult patients with active disease and in remission. Blood 71:709-716, 1988.
3. Lotzová E, Savary CA, Herberman RB: Induction of NK cell activity against fresh human leukemia in culture with Interleukin 2. J Immunol 138:2718-2727, 1987.
4. Oshimi K, Oshimi Y, Akutsu M, et al: Cytotoxicity of Interleukin 2-activated lymphocytes for leukemia and lymphoma cells. Blood 68:938-948, 1986.
5. Allavena P, Damia G, Colombo T, et al: Lymphokine-activated killer (LAK) and monocyte-mediated cytotoxicity on tumor cell lines resistant to antitumor agents. Cell Immunol 120:250-258, 1989.
6. Landay AL, Zarcone D, Grossi CE, et al: Relationship between target cell cycle and susceptibility to natural killer lysis. Cancer Res 47:2767-2770, 1987.
7. Lista P, Fierro MT, Liao X-S, et al: Lymphokine-activated killer (LAK) cells inhibit the clonogenic growth of human leukemic stem cells. Eur J Haematol 42:425-430, 1989.
8. Lotzová E, Savary CA , Herberman RB: Inhibition of clonogenic growth of fresh leukemia cells by unstimulated and IL- 2 stimulated NK cells of normal donors. Leuk Res 11:1059-1066, 1987.
9. Allison MAK, Jones SE, McGuffey P: Phase II trial of outpatient interleukin-2 in malignant lymphoma, chronic lymphocytic leukemia, and selected solid tumors. J Clin Oncol 7:75-80, 1989.
10. Rosenberg SA, Lotze MT, Muul LM, et al: A progress report on the treatment of 157 patients with advanced cancer using lym-

phokine-activated killer cells and interleukin-2 or high-dose interleukin-2 alone. N Engl J Med 316:889-897, 1987.

11. Weber J, Yang J, Topalian S, et al: The use of Interleukin-2 and lymphokine-activated killer cells for the treatment of patients with non-Hodgkin's lymphoma. J Clin Oncol 10:33-40, 1992.

12. West WH, Tauer KW, Yannelli JR, et al: Constant-infusion recombinant interleukin-2 in adoptive immunotherapy of advanced cancer. N Engl J Med 316:898-905, 1987.

13. Foa R, Fierro MT, Tosti S, et al: Induction and persistence of complete remission in a resistant acute myeloid leukemia patient after treatment with recombinant interleukin-2. Leuk and Lymph 1:113-117, 1990.

14. Foa R, Meloni G, Tosti S, et al: Treatment of residual disease in acute leukemia patients with recombinant interleukin 2 (IL2): Clinical and biological findings. Bone Marrow Transplant 6:98-102, 1990.

15. Foa R, Meloni G, Tosti S, et al: Treatment of acute myeloid leukaemia patients with recombinant interleukin 2: A pilot study. Br J Haematol 77:491-496, 1991.

16. Maraninchi D, Blaise D, Viens P, et al: High-dose recombinant Interleukin-2 and acute myeloid leukemias in relapse. Blood 78:2182-2187, 1991.

17. Benyunes MC, Fefer A: IL-2 in the Treatment of Hematologic Malignancies. In M Atkins, J Mier (eds): Therapeutic Applications of Interleukin. Volume 2. New York, NY, Marcel Dekker, 1993, pp 163-175.

18. Massumoto C, Benyunes MC, Sale G, et al: Induction of cutaneous graft-versus-host disease by administration of interleukin-2 after autologous bone marrow transplantation for hematologic malignancy. Blood 80:134a, 1992.

19. Fefer A, Truitt RL, Sullivan KM: Adoptive cellular therapy: Graft-vs-tumor responses after bone marrow transplantation. In V DeVita, S Hellman, S Rosenberg (eds): Biologic Therapy of Cancer: Principles and Practice. Philadelphia, Pa, JB Lippincott Co., 1991, pp 237-246.

20. Bernstein ZP, Vaickus L, Friedman N, et al: IL-2 LAK therapy of non-Hodgkin's lymphoma and Hodgkin's disease. J Immunother 10:141-146, 1991.

21. Gisselbrecht C, Maraninchi D, Pico J, et al: Interleukin 2 (IL2) in lymphoma: A phase II multicentric study. Blood. In press.

22. Margolin K, Aronson F, Sznol M, et al: Phase II trial of high-dose interleukin-2 and lymphokine activated killer cells in Hodgkin's disease and non-Hodgkin's lymphoma. J Immunother 10:214-220, 1991.

23. Schoof DD, Gramolini BA, Davidson DL, et al: Adoptive immunotherapy of human cancer using low-dose recombinant interleukin-2 and lymphokine-activated killer cells. Cancer Res 48:5007-5010, 1988.
24. Tourani J, Levy V, Briere J, et al: Interleukin-2 therapy for refractory and relapsing lymphomas. Eur J Cancer 27:1676-1680, 1991.
25. Paciucci PA, Holland JF, Glidewell O, et al: Recombinant interleukin-2 by continuous infusion and adoptive transfer of recombinant interleukin-2-activated cells in patients with advanced cancer. J Clin Oncol 7:869-878, 1989.
26. Foa R: Does Interleukin-2 have a role in the management of acute leukemia? J Clin Oncol 11:1817-1825, 1933.
27. Archimbaud E, Bailly M, Dore J-F: Inducibility of lymphokine activated killer (LAK) cells in patients with acute myelogenous leukaemia in complete remission and its clinical relevance. Br J Haematol 77:328-334, 1991.
28. Foa R, Fierro M, Raspadori D, et al: Lymphokine-activated killer (LAK) activity in B and T chronic lymphoid leukemia defective LAK generation and reduced susceptibility of the leukemic cells to allogeneic and autologous LAK effectors. Blood 76:1349-1354, 1990.
29. Petersen F, Appelbaum F, Hill R, et al: Autologous marrow transplantation for malignant lymphoma: A report of 101 cases from Seattle. J Clin Oncol 8:638-647, 1990.
30. Petersen FB, Lynch MHE, Clift R, et al: Autologous marrow transplantation for patients with acute myeloid leukemia in untreated first relapse or in second complete remission. J Clin Oncol 11:1353-1360, 1993.
31. Philip T, Armitage J, Spitzer G, et al: High dose therapy and autologous bone marrow transplantation after failure of conventional chemotherapy in adults with intermediate grade or high grade non-Hodgkin's lymphoma. N Engl J Med 316:1493-1498, 1987.
32. Takvorian T, Canellos G, Ritz J, et al: Prolonged disease- free survival after autologous bone marrow transplantation in patients with non-Hodgkin's lymphoma with a poor prognosis. N Engl J Med 316:1499-1505, 1987.
33. Yeager A, Kaizer H, Santos G, et al: Autologous bone marrow transplantation in patients with acute nonlymphocytic leukemia, using *ex vivo* marrow treatment with 4- hydroperoxycyclophosphamide. N Engl J Med 315:142-147, 1986.
34. Blaise D, Viens P, Olive D, et al: Recombinant interleukin 2

(rIL2) after autologous bone marrow transplantation (BMT): A pilot study in 19 patients. Eur Cytokine Net 2:121-129, 1991.

35. Gottlieb DJ, Brenner MK, Heslop HE, et al: A phase I clinical trial of recombinant interleukin 2 following high dose chemo-radiotherapy for haematological malignancy: Applicability to the elimination of minimal residual disease. Br J Cancer 60:610-615, 1989.

36. Heslop H, Bello-Fernandez C, Reittie J, et al: Interleukin 2 infusion after autologous bone marrow transplantation of chemotherapy enhances hemopoietic regeneration. Blood 76:544, 1990. Abstract.

37. Higuchi C, Thompson J, Cox T, et al: Lymphokine-activated killer function following autologous bone marrow transplantation for refractory hematologic malignancies. Cancer Res 49:5509-5513, 1989.

38. Reittie JE, Gottlieb D, Heslop HE, et al: Endogenously generated activated killer cells circulate after autologous and allogeneic marrow transplantation but not after chemotherapy. Blood 73:1351-1358, 1989.

39. Ettinghausen SE, Moore JG, White DE, et al: Hematologic effects of immunotherapy with lymphocyte-activated killer cells and recombinant Interleukin-2 in cancer patients. Blood 69:1654- 1660, 1987.

40. Weisdorf DJ, Anderson PM, Blazar BR, et al: Interleukin 2 immediately after autologous bone marrow transplantation for acute lymphoblastic leukemia—A phase I study. Transplantation 55:61-66.

41. Blaise D, Olive D, Stoppa AM, et al: Hematologic and immunologic effects of the systemic administration of recombinant Interleukin-2 after autologous bone marrow transplantation. Blood 76:1092-1097, 1990.

42. Soiffer R, Murray C, Cochran K, et al: Clinical and Immunologic effects of prolonged infusion of low-dose recombinant interleukin-2 after autologous and T-cell-depleted allogeneic bone marrow transplantation. Blood 79:517-526, 1992.

43. Foa R, Guarini A, Tos AG, et al: Peripheral blood and bone marrow immunophenotypic and functional modifications induced in acute leukemia patients treated with Interleukin 2: Evidence of *in vivo* lymphokine activated killer cell generation. Cancer Res 51:964-968, 1991.

44. Margolin KA, Rayner A, Hawkins MJ, et al: Interleukin-2 and lymphokine-activated killer cell therapy of solid tumors: Analysis of toxicity and management guidelines. J Clin Oncol 7:486-498, 1989.

45. Rosenberg SA, Lotze MT, Yang JC, et al: Experience with the use of high-dose interleukin-2 in the treatment of 652 cancer patients. Ann Surg 210:474-485, 1989.
46. Thompson J, Peace D, Klarnet J, et al: Eradication of disseminated murine leukemia by treatment with high-dose Interleukin 2. J Immunol 137:3675-3680, 1986.
47. Blaise D, Stoppa A, Brandelys M, et al: Treatment of relapsed acute myeloid leukemia (AML) with systemic recombinant Interleukin 2 (IL2). Blood 76:255, 1990. Abstract.
48. Heslop H, Duncombe A, Reittie J, et al: Interleukin 2 infusion induces haemopoietic growth factors and modifies marrow regeneration after chemotherapy or autologous marrow transplantation. Br J Haematol 77:237-244, 1991.
49. MacDonald D, Gordon A, Kajitani H, et al: Interleukin-2 treatment-associated eosinophilia is mediated by interleukin-5 production. Br J Haematol 76:168-173, 1990.
50. Higuchi CM, Thompson JA, Petersen FB, et al: Toxicity and immunomodulatory effects of Interleukin 2 after autologous bone marrow transplantation for hematologic malignancies. Blood 77:2561-2568, 1991.
51. Thompson JA, Lee DJ, Lindgren CG, et al: Influence of schedule of interleukin 2 administration on therapy with interleukin 2 and lymphokine activated killer cells. Cancer Res 49:235-240, 1989.
52. Fefer A, Benyunes M, Massumoto C, et al: Interleukin-2 therapy after autologous bone marrow transplantation for hematological malignancies. Seminars in Oncology 20(6):41-45, 1993.
53. Benyunes M, Massumoto C, Higuchi C, et al: Interleukin-2+/-lymphokine-activated killer cells as consolidative immunotherapy after autologous bone marrow transplantation for acute myelogenous leukemia: A preliminary report. Bone Marrow Transplant 12:159-163, 1993.
54. Benyunes M, York A, Lindgren C, et al: IL-2± LAK cells as consolidative therapy after autologous BMT for hematologic malignancies: A feasibility trial. Proc Am Soc Clin Oncol 11:319, 1992. Abstract.
55. Chao N, Schriber J, Grimes K, et al: Granulocyte colony- stimulating factor "mobilized" peripheral blood progenitor cells accelerate granulocyte and platelet recovery after high-dose chemotherapy. Blood 81:2031-2035, 1993.
56. Neubauer M, Benyunes M, Thompson J, et al: Lymphokine- activated killer (LAK) precursor cell activity is present in infused peripheral blood stem cells and in the blood after autologous pe-

ripheral blood stem cell transplantation. Bone Marrow Transplant 13:311-316, 1994.

57. Higuchi C, Triesman J, Thompson J, et al: Cytolytic T- lymphocytes infiltrating human melanoma expanded by culture with interleukin-2. Proc Am Asso Cancer Res 31:269, 1990. Abstract.

58. Chopra R, Goldstone A, McMillan A, et al: Successful treatment of acute myeloid leukemia beyond first remission with autologous bone marrow transplantation using busulfan/cyclophosphamide and unpurged marrow: The British Autograft Group experience. J Clin Oncol 9:1840-1847, 1991.

59. Gorin N, Aegerter P, Auvert B, et al: Autologous bone marrow transplantation for acute myelocytic leukemia in first remission: A European survey of the role of marrow purging. Blood 75:1606-1614, 1990.

60. Stewart P, Buckner C, Bensinger W, et al: Autologous marrow transplantation in patients with acute nonlymphocytic leukemia in first remission. Exp Hematol 13:267-272, 1985.

61. Clift R, Buckner C, Thomas E, et al: The treatment of acute non-lymphoblastic leukemia by allogeneic marrow transplantation. Bone Marrow Transplant 2:243-258, 1987.

62. Pavletic Z, Benyunes M, Thompson J, et al: Induction by interleukin-7 of lymphokine-activated killer activity in lymphocytes from autologous and syngeneic marrow transplant recipients before and after systemic interleukin-2 therapy. Exp Hematol 12:1371-1378, 1993.

63. Soiffer R, Robertson M, Murray C, et al: Interleukin-12 augments cytolytic activity of peripheral blood lymphocytes from patients with hematologic and solid malignancies. Blood 82:2790-2796, 1993.

64. Cheever M, Greenberg P, Fefer A, et al: Augmentation of the anti-tumor therapeutic efficacy of long-term cultured T lymphocytes by *in vivo* administration of purified Interleukin-2. J Exp Med 155:968-980, 1982.

65. Cheever M, Chen W, Nelson H, et al: T cell immunity to the oncogenic form of *ras* protein can be induced by immunization with synthetic peptides. In M Lotze, O Finn (eds): Cellular Immunity and Immunotherapy of Cancer. New York, NY, Wiley-Liss, Inc., 1990, pp 295-302.

66. Peace D, Chen W, Nelson H, et al: T cell recognition of transforming proteins encoded by mutated ras proto-oncogenes. J Immunol 146:2059-2065, 1991.

67. Chen W, Peace D, Rovira D, et al: T cell immunity to the joining region of p210 bcr-abl protein. Proc Natl Acad Sci U S A 89:1468-1472, 1992.

68. Gedde-Dahl T III, Spurkland A, Eriksen JA, et al: Memory T cells of a patient with follicular thyroid carcinoma recognize peptides derived from mutated p21 *ras* (Gln→Leu61). Int J Immunother 4:1331-1337, 1992.

69. Cheever MA, Chen W, Disis ML, et al: T-cell immunity to oncogenic proteins including mutated *ras* and chimeric bcr-abl. In J-C Bystryn, S Ferrone, P Livingston (eds): Specific Immunotherapy of Cancer with Vaccines. New York, NY, New York Academy of Sciences, 1993, pp 101-112.

70. Chen W, You S, Disis M, et al: Evaluation of the joining region segment of p210[BCR-ABL] chimeric protein as a potential leukemia-specific antigen to elicit class I MHC-restricted CTL responses. J Cell Biochem 17D(Suppl):107, 1993.

71. Gedde-Dahl T III, Olsen BH, Thorsby E, Guadernack G: Oncogene-derived peptides: A new class of tumor rejection antigens? Transplant Proc 25:1385-1386, 1993.

72. Disis ML, Smith JW, Murphy AE, et al: *In vitro* generation of human cytotoxic T cells specific for peptides derived from the HER-2/*neu* proto-oncogene protein. Cancer Res 54 (4):1071-1076, 1994.

73. Peace DJ, Smith JW, Disis ML, et al: Induction of T cells specific for the mutated segment of oncogenic p21[ras] protein by immunization *in vivo* with the oncogenic protein. J Immunother 14:110-114, 1993.

74. Ioannides C, Ioannides M, O'Brian C: T cell recognition of oncogene products: A new strategy for immunotherapy. Mol Carcinogenesis 6:77-82, 1992.

75. Ioannides CG, Fisk B, Fan D, et al: Cytotoxic T cells isolated from ovarian malignant ascites recognize a peptide derived from the HER-2/neu proto-oncogene. Cell Immunol 151:225- 234, 1993.

76. Yanuck M, Carbone D, Pendleton C, et al: A mutant p53 tumor suppressor protein is a target for peptide-induced CD8 and cytotoxic T-cells. Cancer Res 53:3257-3261, 1993.

77. Riddell S, Watanabe K, Goodrich J, et al: Restoration of viral immunity in immunocompromised humans by the adoptive transfer of T cell clones. Science 257:238-241, 1992.

Chapter 7

Interferons As Immunotherapeutic Agents After Marrow Transplantation

Hans-G Klingemann, M.D., Ph.D., M.J. Barnett, B.M., T. Kuhr, M.D.

Bone marrow transplantation (BMT) is widely used to treat various hematological diseases and some selected solid tumors.[1] After an allogeneic BMT, immune mechanisms triggered by alloantigen recognizing donor T lymphocytes can contribute to the elimination of residual malignant clonogenic cells.[2,3] This graft-versus-leukemia/lymphoma (GVL) effect often occurs in the context of acute graft-versus-host disease (GVHD) and includes a release of antiproliferative cytokines, such as interferon (IFN) and tumor necrosis factor (TNF)-α.[4] A significant GVL effect probably does not occur after autologous (or syngeneic) transplantation, and any malignant cells that were not eliminated by high-dose chemotherapy/irradiation or have been infused with the marrow inoculum can potentially cause relapse.[5]

Recently, a number of immunotherapeutic approaches using either cell preparations (eg, buffy coat (BC)[6,7]) or cytokines[8] have been utilized based on their ability to prevent disease recurrence, particularly after autologous or T-lymphocyte-depleted allogeneic BMT.

From: Spitzer T, Mazumder A: Immunotherapy and Bone Marrow Transplantation. Armonk, NY, Futura Publishing Co., Inc., © 1995.

Among the cytokines, interleukin (IL)-2 and IFN-α have been studied in the first clinical trials to date.[9-12] In the nontransplant setting, the antiproliferative and immunomodulatory abilities of IFNs have resulted in disease control in a proportion of patients with chronic myeloid leukemia (CML), hairy-cell leukemia, multiple myeloma (MM) and non-Hodgkin's lymphoma (NHL).[13-21] These have led to the conclusion that IFNs should have even more efficacy in situations where malignant cells have been reduced to a "minimal disease" state, such as after BMT. Here we review the emerging field of in vivo studies that describe the use of IFNs as immunotherapeutic agents to prevent relapse after marrow transplantation.

Mechanism of Action of Interferons

IFNs can be classified according to their biochemical characteristics into three major subtypes, designated IFN-α, IFN-β, and IFN-γ. Among the spectrum of biological properties, their immunoregulatory and antiproliferative effects have been of major interest. IFNs regulate the growth and differentiation of both normal and tumor cells. These effects can be mediated via induction and inhibition of proteins of which major histocompatibility complex (MHC) antigens are the best characterized. Host cells constitutively express MHC antigens in vivo, which can be markedly enhanced upon stimulation with IFNs.[22] MHC Class I antigens are also involved in the recognition of non-self antigens by cytotoxic T-lymphocytes (CTL). Tumor cells can express specific antigens, but it is believed that their ability to present these antigens in the context of MHC Class I antigens may be poor, due to a low basal level of such antigens. Thus, by enhancing expression of MHC Class I antigen, IFNs may be able to indirectly "stimulate" the host defense against clonogenic cells. Moreover, in vitro studies[22] and clinical trials of tumor patients[23] have suggested that IFN treatment can result in augmented expression of tumor-associated antigen on the surface of tumor cells.

Oncogenes participate in the regulation of cell growth during the early stages, and have also been associated with the growth of malignant cells once they become activated. IFNs can decrease the expression of proto-oncogenes such as c-myc.[24] Some hematological malignancies are associated with a loss of IFN genes, suggesting a possible involvement of IFNs as tumor-suppressor genes in leukemia.[25]

The antiproliferative effect of IFNs could also be mediated through the induction of the RNA-dependent protein, kinase (p68).[26] Induced by IFNs and activated by double-stranded RNA, this kinase terminates protein synthesis by phosphorylating the eukaryotic initiation factor 2 (eIF2). Hence, enhanced expression of this enzyme by IFN treatment could be inhibitory to malignant cell growth.

Synergistic effects of IFNs with other cytokines, such as IL-2 and TNF-α have been described.[27] For example, IFN-γ can induce receptors for TNF-α,[28,29] rendering tumor cells more susceptible to the cytotoxic and/or cytostatic effects of TNF-α.

Immunoregulatory functions of IFN relate to its ability to enhance the function of monocytes, neutrophils, and natural killer (NK) cells. The mechanisms by which IFNs act on the activity of NK cells is not completely known. They can increase the expression of IL-2 receptors on NK progenitor cells and enhance the lytic activity of already activated cells. They also provide a "bypass" to the inhibitory effect of prostaglandin E_2 (PGE$_2$) which can be produced by tumor cells and suppressor macrophages.[30] Upon activation with IFNs, NK cells become partially resistant to suppression by PGE$_2$.

Unlike NK cells, macrophages normally exhibit low spontaneous cytotoxicity. However, upon stimulation with IFN-γ, they can develop into cytotoxic effector cells which can mediate "nonspecific" tumor cell lysis.[31] In addition, IFN-γ can also prime monocytes/macrophages to produce TNF-α, as well as IL-1, which can enhance the secretion of IL-2 and its receptor.[32] The generation of various CTL populations including tumor-infiltrating lymphocytes (TIL) and cytokine-activated natural killer (A-NK) cells may then lead to an amplified cytolytic response.

The emergence of neutralizing antibodies against IFN has been correlated with hematological relapse in patients with CML,[33,34] hairy-cell leukemia,[35] and some malignant tumors.[36] It is more frequently observed with recombinant IFN preparations, whereas antibody formation against natural IFN seems to be negligible.[37] There is also evidence that clinical responses can be achieved by changing from recombinant IFN to natural IFN.[34] It is unlikely that significant specific antibody production occurs in immunocompromised marrow transplant recipients, especially during short-term treatment. No neutralizing antibodies were found in the serum of patients treated for 2 months with IFN-α2b early after BMT.[10] However, in situations where long-term treatment is preferred, possibility of antibody formation must be considered.

Clinical Experience with Interferon-α after Autologous Bone Marrow Transplantation

Treatment with IFN-α can result in durable hematological and cytogenetic remissions in CML,[15,21] and induce and prolong responses in MM[16,18] and low-grade NHL.[19,20] Such observations serve as a rationale for the use of IFN-α as maintenance treatment in these diseases after intensive therapy requiring autologous hematopoietic stem cell rescue.

The Bordeaux group treated a subset of patients who had transformed CML with intensive therapy and autografting on two occasions: the first, to reestablish chronic phase; followed by the second, as consolidation.[38] After recovery from the second autograft, IFN-α 5×10^6 U/m^2 three times a week was given without significant toxicity. Eleven of 17 patients received the full treatment as intended. The relative contribution of the components of the treatment, ie, double autografting and IFN-α maintenance, is not possible to determine. Nevertheless, the median duration of the second chronic phase for all 17 patients was 18 months, which suggests that the overall strategy was an effective one. Indeed, on the basis of this result, the group has proposed to employ this program in patients with chronic phase CML.

In a pilot study, we have used a 10-day cultured marrow autograft to support intensive treatment of patients with either chronic phase or transformed CML.[39,40] In 13 of 22 selected patients, complete (morphological and cytogenetic) remission was achieved. However, some Philadelphia chromosome (Ph)-positive cells reappeared between 4 and 36 months postautograft in all but 1 of the 13 patients; the remaining patient died in remission. Nine of these 12 patients were then treated with IFN-α 1 to 3×10^6 U/m^2 three to seven times a week. Four subsequently returned to complete remission, 3 developed increasing numbers of Ph-positive cells, and 2 are too early to evaluate. Overall, toxicity from IFN-α was mild. Encouraged by these results, a revised protocol has been initiated which involves the administration of IFN-α (1×10^6 U/m^2, increasing to 3×10^6 U/m^2, three times a week) early postautograft, once hematological recovery has occurred.

Other groups[41,42] have reported the use of IFN-α early postautografting for chronic phase CML. In most of these patients, it is not possible to determine whether the natural history of the disease was altered by this treatment. It is, however, interesting to note that in the series from the M.D. Anderson Cancer Center,[42] three of seven patients, in whom hematological resistance to IFN-α had been documented before the autograft, had evidence of responsive disease following the autograft. Thus, intensive therapy and autografting in patients with chronic phase CML may induce sensitivity to IFN-α in those previously resistant to it.

The Royal Marsden/St. Bartholomew's group has conducted a randomized trial of maintenance IFN-α after intensive therapy and marrow autografting in MM.[43] After induction therapy followed by high-dose melphalan and autografting as consolidation, 84 patients were randomized to receive either IFN-α 3×10^6 U/m^2 three times a week, or no treatment. At a median follow-up of 24 months, the IFN-α group had a significantly longer median progression-free survival than the control group (39 months versus 27 months). For the subset of patients (n=62) in whom complete remission was achieved after high dose melphalan, remission was significantly prolonged in the IFN-α group (53% remain in remission 4 years postautograft). In contrast, those in whom complete remission was not achieved did achieve benefit from IFN-α.

In a prospective, nonrandomized study, the Toulouse group gave maintenance IFN-α to patients with MM after autografting.[44] The protocol included induction followed by consolidation with high-dose melphalan/total body irradiation (TBI) and marrow autografting. IFN-α at 3×10^6 U/m^2 three times a week was begun once hematological recovery had occurred following the autograft and was well tolerated. The overall survival from diagnosis for the whole group (n=35) was 81% at 3.5 years postautograft. The probability of progression-free survival at 33 months postautograft was significantly better for patients in whom complete remission was achieved than those in whom it had not (85% versus 24%).

In conclusion, these studies suggest that IFN-α 3×10^6 U/m^2 three times a week following autografting for CML and MM is well-tolerated and effective in maintaining remissions. Studies are also underway in NHL.[45]

Clinical Experience with Interferon-α after Allogeneic Bone Marrow Transplantation

The first and, so far, only randomized study with IFN-α after allogeneic BMT was published in 1988 by Meyers and colleagues, from

Seattle.[46] The initial intent of that trial was to evaluate the efficacy of IFN-α in decreasing the incidence of cytomegalovirus (CMV) disease in a group of children after allogeneic BMT for acute lymphoblastic leukemia (ALL). Patients were randomized either to receive or not receive 6×10^4 U/kg per day of natural leukocyte IFN for 2 to 3 months after allogeneic BMT. The surprising finding was that IFN did not affect the incidence of CMV disease, but patients in the IFN treatment group had a significantly lower leukemic relapse rate (36% versus 74%). No increase in the incidence of acute GVHD was seen. However, the investigators felt that some neurological side effects (encephalopathy, seizures) that occurred in the treatment group might have been related to IFN. On the other hand, a higher percentage of patients in the treatment group had recent cranial irradiation which could either, on its own, explain the increased incidence of neurological complications, or lower the threshhold for severe central nervous system (CNS) effects of IFN.

In a Phase I study with recombinant IFN-α in patients after autologous or allogeneic BMT, we did not encounter any such side effects.[10] IFN, in this study, was commenced within 3 months after marrow grafting once an absolute neutrophil count of $>2 \times 10^9$/L and a platelet count of $>50 \times 10^9$/L had been reached. Contrary to the study from Seattle, we were unable to escalate the dose of IFN-α beyond 1×10^6/m² per day because of marrow suppression (neutropenia and thrombocytopenia). Furthermore, we observed 3 of 11 allogeneic patients in whom IFN-α very likely had induced acute GVHD which promptly responded to steroid treatment. IFN—induced GVHD was also suspected in a patient reported from another center.[47] Patients in our study experienced mostly constitutional symptoms such as fevers, headaches, malaise, and lack of appetite.

IFN-α therapy for patients with Ph¹-positive CML who have relapsed after unmanipulated[48-50] or T-lymphocyte-depleted[51] allogeneic BMT has led to hematologic and/or cytogenetic remission in a certain proportion of patients. Higano et al.[48] administered IFN-α2b to 18 patients with CML who had relapsed cytogenetically and hematologically into chronic phase after unmanipulated BMT. The initial IFN-α dose was 3×10^6 U/m² per day, which was escalated to the maximum tolerated dose of 6×10^6 U/m² per day. IFN normalized the white cell count in all but 2 patients, and also controlled the platelet count in 6 of 6 patients. In 33% of the patients, the Ph¹-clone disappeared and 11% had a partial response as defined by a reduction to ≤35% Ph¹-positive metaphases. There was no response after 9 to 12 months of therapy with IFN-α in 28% of the patients, and 22% progressed to accelerated phase or blast crisis. Treatment of these patients continued for at least 6 months and those who responded were given IFN-α at a maintenance dose of 1.5×10^6 U/m² three times a week for at least 1 year. Although the number of patients is small, it appeared that cytogenetic "responders" had relapsed earlier after BMT and were thus placed on IFN-α sooner after BMT than cytogenetic "nonresponders". It is notable that 8 of the 18 patients in this study had aggressive disease, since 3 had received a BMT in accelerated phase; 3, in blast crisis; and 2, after a second BMT. Severe side effects of IFN-α were seen in 6 patients consisting of fatigue, weight loss, nausea, vomiting, diarrhea, confusion and depression. One patient developed signs of chronic GVHD after starting IFN-α on day 72 after BMT.

In another study, IFN-α2b, at a dose of 5×10^6 U/m², was given three times a week to patients with relapse after T-cell-depleted (TCD) marrow transplant for CML.[51] Four patients had hematological relapse, and 14 had cytogenetic relapse. All 4 patients with hematological relapse achieved a long-lasting remission with reduction of Ph¹-positive cells. Two of 14 patients with cytogenetic relapse achieved complete remission with disappearance of the rearranged bcr band (by Southern blotting) after 6 and 10 months of IFN-α treatment, respectively. Although there was good evidence that these 2 responding patients did have persistence of the Ph¹-clone, it is also true that spontaneous cytogenetic remissions in CML have been reported.[52] In the study by Arcese et al.,[51] IFN-α had to be discontinued or the dose lowered in 38% of patients on treatment because of side effects, and the overall daily dose (mean: ±SD) of IFN-α in all patients was 1.66 ± 0.5 U/m².

Aside from its marrow suppressive side effect, IFN-α may also induce graft rejection. This has been reported in occasional patients after renal transplantation,[53,54] and in one patient after allogeneic BMT for paroxysmal nocturnal hemoglobinuria, who had received IFN-α for the treatment of chronic active hepatitis.[55]

The general conclusion from these studies is that IFN-α has substantial marrow suppressive effects when given within the first few months after allogeneic BMT. It is effective in inducing complete responses in some patients after recurrence of CML after allogeneic BMT. Responses seem to occur in a similar proportion of patients who receive IFN-α for newly diagnosed CML, and it appears that lower doses are required to control the disease when given after BMT. It may be speculated that in addition to the antiproliferative effects of IFN-α, an increased expression of MHC-antigen and/or the bcr-abl gene product as target structure for allogeneic T cells could contribute to the activity of IFN-α in CML. Thus far, no studies have been reported using IFN-α to prevent relapse after BMT for acute myeloid leukemia (AML) and/or myelodysplastic syndrome (MDS).

Interferon-α as Part of Combined Immunotherapeutic Approaches

Interferon-α and Buffy Coat Infusions After Allogeneic Bone Marrow Transplantation

BC infusions can induce reversal to complete donor chimerism in patients who experience a cytogenetic or hematologic relapse after allogeneic transplantation for CML.[6,56] IFN-α given prior to BC infusions may help to "debulk" the malignant cell burden, and may also induce and/or enhance MHC expression on leukemic cells as potential target structures for BC-lymphocytes.[6] Since IFN-α itself can induce GVHD,[10,57] its use, in conjunction with BC, would be expected to also increase any GVL-like activity of BC infusions, assuming GVHD and GVL-reactions are interrelated. However, the clinical data, as yet, do not clearly suggest such a benefit of the addition of IFN-α and more results, ideally in a prospective study, will be helpful to determine the role, if any, of IFN-α in this combination.

Interferon-α and Cyclosporine in the Induction of Autologous Graft-Versus-Host Disease

Cyclosporine (CsA), when given at low doses for about 4 weeks after autologous BMT, can induce autologous GVHD which is usually self-limited and rarely affects organs other than the skin.[58,59] The potential GVL effect is seen in the suppression of malignant cells by autoreactive lymphocytes that react with target cells bearing MHC Class II antigens.[60,61] Studies in a rat model have shown that preincubation of tumor target cells with IFN-γ significantly increased MHC Class II expression, and augmented lysis by syngeneic effector cells. Rats receiving both CsA and IFN-γ developed an enhanced antitumor effect.[62] Clinical trials with the combination of IFN-α and CsA have been initiated to define the optimal dose of IFN-α, and toxicities of the combined treatment early after marrow infusion.[57] CsA (1 mg/kg) was given by continuous infusion for 28 days together with different doses of IFN-α2a (1×10^6 U per day and 3×10^6 U per day). Side effects at the higher IFN-dose level were significant, including intractable nausea, vomiting, severe fatigue, high fever and respiratory distress necessitating discontinuation of IFN in three of four patients. Since this was a Phase I study, no conclusions about the antitumor effect of this approach could be derived. Interestingly, IFN-α induced a rash in some patients that histologically closely resembled acute GVHD.

Interferon-α in Combination with Interleukin-2

IFN-2 or IL-2, although through different mechanisms, can inhibit leukemia cell growth.[27] This has triggered clinical trials in which the cytokines are given either concomitantly or sequentially. In an ongoing study in Jerusalem, patients with lymphoma and leukemia after engraftment are receiving IFN-α at a dose of 3×10^6 U/m^2 per day subcutaneously (s.c.) on 5 of 7 weekdays for 2 months, with a 1-month break in-between. IL-2 at 10^6 U/m^2 per day is given on the same schedule. Results of this and similar studies are pending (S. Slavin, personal communication).

Clinical Experience with Interferon-γ after Bone Marrow Transplantation

IFN-γ production appears to be low after BMT even in recipients who do not have GVHD and are not receiving immunosuppressive medications.[63] The cytokine, on the other hand, has potent immunoregulatory abilities that would make it a candidate for posttransplant immunostimulation. Moreover, it has been demonstrated that IFN-γ can induce monocytic differentiation of blast cells from patients with AML and MDS.[64] From studies in CML patients, it is anticipated that there could be more side effects than seen with comparable doses of IFN-α (Table 1).[65,66] Only one clinical study in marrow recipients has been presented in abstract form.[67] IFN-γ was given in combination with IL-2 and toxicities were substantial. Animal data suggest that IFN-γ can potentiate the antitumor effect of CsA-induced autoimmunity.[62] One obvious concern with its use after allogeneic BMT is its potential to induce or aggravate acute GVHD through up-regulation of the expression of minor MHC antigens.

Although IFN-γ is generally considered "marrow-toxic," in vitro data suggests that it can enhance normal colony formation, particularly when hematopoietic growth factors are present.[68]

Table 1
Summary of Side Effects of IFN-α in Marrow Transplant Patients

---

Fever

Malaise

Headache

Weight loss

Nausea, vomiting

Joint pain

Diarrhea

Neurological symptoms

    mental depression
    loss of memory
    seizures

Hepatic toxicity

Marrow toxicity with

    granulocytopenia
    thrombocytopenia
    anemia

Exacerbation of acute graft vs host disease

Graft rejection

IFN-α: Interferon- alpha

Future Directions

Because of their systemic side effects when given early after BMT, it would be desirable to have IFNs released site-specific in the bone marrow (BM) where minimal residual leukemia generally resides. Such a strategy of targeted cytokine therapy has been shown to activate immune cells locally.[69] Aerosolized IFN-γ activated pulmonary macrophages locally but had no systemic side effects. A similar rationale forms the basis for using retroviral gene transfer of IFN-γ and other immunomodulatory cytokines into more committed hematopoietic progenitor cells which could be infused together with unmanipulated marrow or peripheral blood progenitor cells. These cells are also expected to home to the marrow and produce IFN locally. One major concern with this treatment, namely suppression of hematopoiesis, might in fact not occur.[68] There is also a concern to insert genes into marrow-derived cells, as "random transduction" of stem cells could occur with as yet unknown consequences.

Immunotherapy after BMT has already become an integral part of the treatment plan at many transplant centers after both autologous and allogeneic BMT. IFNs represent only one group of cytokines with antileukemic and antiproliferative activity which will likely be most useful in conjunction with other non-chemo- radiotherapeutic approaches aimed at overcoming residual disease.[8]

Acknowledgments: The authors wish to thank Toni Jewall and Linda Williams for assistance in manuscript preparation.

References

1. Thomas ED: Adolfo Ferrata Lecture 1991. Bone marrow transplantation: Past, present and future. Haematologica 76:353-356, 1991.
2. Weiden PL, Flournoy N, Thomas ED, et al: Antileukemic effect of graft-versus-host disease in human recipients of allogeneic marrow grafts. N Engl J Med 300:1068-1073, 1979.
3. Horowitz MM, Gale RP, Sondel PM, et al: Graft-versus-leukemia reactions after bone marrow transplantation. Blood 75:555-562, 1990.
4. Antin JH, Ferrara JLM: Cytokine dysregulation and acute graft-versus-host disease. Blood 80:2964-2968, 1992.
5. Brenner MK, Rill DR, Moen RC, et al: Gene-marking to trace origin of relapse after autologous bone-marrow transplantation. Lancet 341:85-86, 1993.
6. Kolb HJ, Mittermuller J, Clemm C, et al: Donor leukocyte transfusions for treatment of recurrent chronic myelogenous leukemia in marrow transplant patients. Blood 76:2462-2465, 1990.
7. Porter DL, Roth M, McGarigle C, et al: Induction of graft- v-leukemia (GvL) with interferon-α (IFN-α) and donor lymphocyte infusions is effective therapy for patients with relapsed CML following allogeneic bone marrow transplant. Blood 80:137a, 1992.
8. Klingemann H-G: Trying to overcome residual disease after bone marrow transplantation for hematologic malignancies. Leuk and Lymph 8:421-429, 1992.

9. Klingemann H-G, Phillips GL: Immunotherapy after bone marrow transplantation. Bone Marrow Transplant 8:73-81, 1991.

10. Klingemann H-G, Grigg AP, Wilkie-Boyd K, et al: Treatment with recombinant interferon (α-2b) early after bone marrow transplantation in patients at high risk for relapse. Blood 78:3306-3311, 1991.

11. Blaise D, Olive D, Stoppa AM, et al: Hematologic and immunologic effects of the systemic administration of recombinant interleukin-2 after autologous bone marrow transplantation. Blood 76:1092-1097, 1990.

12. Higuchi CM, Thompson JA, Petersen FB, et al: Toxicity and immunomodulatory effects of interleukin-2 after autologous bone marrow transplantation for hematologic malignancies. Blood 77:2561-2568, 1991.

13. Balkwill FR: Interferons. Lancet 1:1060-1063, 1989.

14. Gutterman JN: The role of interferons in the treatment of hematologic malignancies. Semin Hematol 25(Suppl 3):3-8, 1988.

15. Talpaz M, Kantarjian H, Kurzrock R, et al: Interferon-alpha produces sustained cytogenetic responses in chronic myelogenous leukemia. Ann Intern Med 114:532-538, 1991.

16. Mandelli F, Avvisati G, Amadori S, et al: Maintenance treatment with recombinant interferon alpha-2b in patients with multiple myeloma responding to conventional induction chemotherapy. N Engl J Med 322:1430-1434, 1990.

17. Smalley RV, Andersen JW, Hawkins MJ, et al: Interferon alpha combined with cytotoxic chemotherapy for patients with non-Hodgkin's lymphoma. N Engl J Med 327:1336-1341, 1992.

18. Quesada JR, Alexanian R, Hawkins M, et al: Treatment of multiple myeloma with recombinant α-interferon. Blood 67:275-278, 1986.

19. Wagstaff J, Loynds P, Crowther D: A phase II study of human rDNA alpha-2 interferon in patients with low grade non-Hodgkin's lymphoma. Cancer Chemother Pharmacol 18:54-58, 1986.

20. Hagenbeek A, Carde P, Somers R, et al: Maintenance of remission with human recombinant alpha-2 interferon (roferon-A) in patients with stages III and IV low grade malignant non-Hodgkin's lymphoma. Results from a prospective, randomised phase III clinical trial in 331 patients. Blood 80(Suppl 1):74a, 1992.

21. Zuffa E: A prospective study of interferon alpha-2A vs chemotherapy in chronic myeloid leukemia (CML): Karyotypic response and survival. Proc Am Soc Clin Oncol 12:300, 1993.

22. Giacomini P, Aguzzi A, Pestka S, et al: Modulation by recombinant DNA leukocyte (α) and fibroblast (β) interferons of the expression and shedding of HLA- and tumor-associated antigens by human melanoma cells. J Immunol 133:1649-1655, 1984.

23. Rosenblum MG, Lamki LM, Murrary JL, et al: Interferon- induced changes in pharmacokinetics and tumor uptake of ^{111}In-labeled antimelanoma antibody 96.5 in melanoma patients. J Natl Cancer Inst 80:160-165, 1988.

24. Dani CH, Mechti N, Piechacyk M, et al: Increased rate of degradation of c-myc mRNA in interferon-treated Daudi cells. Proc Natl Acad Sci U S A 82:4896-4899, 1985.

25. Diaz MO, Ziemin S, LeBeau MM, et al: Homozygous deletion of the α and β1-interferon genes in human leukemia and derived cell lines. Proc Natl Acad Sci U S A 85:5229-5263, 1988.

26. Meuers EF, Galabru J, Barber GN, et al: Tumor suppressor function of the interferon-induced double-stranded RNA-activated protein kinase. Proc Natl Acad Sci U S A 90:232-236, 1992.

27. Herberman RB, Ernstoff MS, Kirkwood JM: Interferon alpha in combination with other biologics: The scientific rationale. Br J Haematol 79(Suppl 1):78-80, 1991.

28. Tsujimoto M, Yip YK, Vilcek J: Interferon γ enhances expression of cellular receptors for tumour necrosis factor. J Immunol 136:2441-2444, 1986.

29. Ruggiero V, Tavernter V, Fiers, W, et al: Induction of the synthesis of tumour necrosis factor receptors by interferon γ. J Immunol 136:2445-2450, 1986.

30. Browning JL, Ribolini A: Interferon blocks interleukin 1- induced prostaglandin release from human peripheral monocytes. J Immunol 138:2857-2863, 1987.

31. Kleinerman ES, Kurzrock R, Wyatt D, et al: Activation or suppression of the tumoricidal properties of monocytes from cancer patients following treatment with human recombinant gamma-interferon. Cancer Res 46:5401-5405, 1986.

32. Kohn FR, Phillips GL, Klingemann H-G: Regulation of tumor necrosis factor-α production and gene expression in monocytes. Bone Marrow Transplant 9:369-376, 1992.

33. Freund M, von Wussow P, Diedrich H, et al: Recombinant human interferon (IFN) alpha-2b in chronic myelogenous leukaemia: Dose dependency of response and frequency of neutralizing anti- interferon antibodies. Br J Haematol 72:350-356, 1989.

34. von Wussow P, Jakschies D, Freund M, et al: Treatment of anti-recombinant interferon-alpha 2 antibody positive CML patients with natural interferon-alpha. Br J Haematol 78:210-216, 1991.

35. Steis RG, Smith JW II, Urba WJ, et al: Resistance to recombinant interferon alpha-2a in hairy-cell leukemia associated with neutralizing anti-interferon antibodies. N Engl J Med 318:1409-1413, 1988.

36. Oberg K, Alm G, Magnusson A, et al: Treatment of malignant carcinoid tumors with recombinant interferon alpha-2b: Development of neutralizing interferon antibodies and possible loss of antitumor activity. J Natl Cancer Inst 81:531-535, 1989.

37. Antonelli G, Currenti M, Turriziani O, et al: Neutralizing antibodies to interferon-α: Relative frequency in patients treated with different interferon preparations. J Infect Dis 163:882-885, 1991.

38. Reiffers J, Trouette R, Marit G, et al: Autologous blood stem cell transplantation for chronic granulocytic leukaemia in transformation: A report of 47 cases. Br J Haematol 77:339-345, 1991.

39. Barnett MJ, Eaves CJ, Phillips GL, et al: Successful autografting in chronic myeloid leukaemia after maintenance of marrow in culture. Bone Marrow Transplant 4:345-351, 1989.

40. Barnett MJ, Eaves CJ, Phillips GL, et al: Autografting in chronic myeloid leukemia with cultured marrow. Leukemia 6(Suppl 4):118-119, 1992.

41. De Fabritiis P, Sandrelli A, Meloni G, et al: Prolonged suppression of myeloid progenitor cell numbers after stopping interferon treatment for CML may necessitate delay in harvesting marrow cells for autografting. Bone Marrow Transplant 6:247-251, 1990.

42. Kantarjian HM, Talpaz M, LeMaistre CF, et al: Intensive combination chemotherapy and autologous bone marrow transplantation leads to the reappearance of Philadelphia chromosome-negative cells in chronic myelogenous leukemia. Cancer 67:2959-2965, 1991.

43. Cunningham D, Powles R, Malpas JS, et al: A randomised trial of maintenance therapy with Intron-A following high dose melphalan and ABMT in myeloma. Proc Am Soc Clin Oncol 12:364, 1993.

44. Attal M, Huguet F, Schlaifer D, et al: Intensive combined therapy for previously untreated myeloma. Blood 79:1130-1136, 1992.

45. Ascensao JL, Miller KB, Tuck D, et al: Immunotherapy with recombinant human interferon alpha 2B (IFN) following autologous bone marrow transplantation (ABMT) for lymphomas: An update. Proc Am Soc Clin Oncol 12:380, 1993.

46. Meyers JD, Flournoy N, Sanders JE, et al: Prophylactic use of human leukocyte interferon after allogeneic marrow transplantation. Ann Intern Med 107:809-816, 1987.

47. Pavord S, Sivakumaran M, Durrant S, et al: The role of alpha interferon in the pathogenesis of GVHD. Bone Marrow Transplant 10:477, 1992.

48. Higano CS, Raskind WH, Singer JW: Use of α interferon for the treatment of relapse of chronic myelogenous leukemia in chronic phase after allogeneic bone marrow transplantation. Blood 80:1437-1442, 1992.

49. Borgies P, Ferrant A, Delannoy A, et al: Interferon alpha induced and maintained complete remission in chronic granulocytic leukemia in relapse after bone marrow transplantation. Bone Marrow Transplant 4:127-128, 1989.

50. Steegmann JL, Perez M, Vasquez L, et al: Interferon alpha treatment of accelerated-phase chronic myeloid leukemia in relapse after bone marrow transplantation: A case with complete cytogenetic and molecular remission. Bone Marrow Transplant 7:65-67, 1991.

51. Arcese W, Mauro FR, Alimena G, et al: Interferon therapy for Ph[1] positive CML patients relapsing after T cell-depleted allogeneic bone marrow transplantation. Bone Marrow Transplant 5:309-315, 1990.

52. Frassoni F, Sessarego M, Bacigalupo A, et al: Competition between recipient and donor cells after bone marrow transplantation for chronic myeloid leukaemia. Br J Haematol 69:471-475, 1988.

53. Kramer P, Bijnen AB, ten Kate FWJ, et al: Recombinant leucocyte interferon A induces steroid-resistant acute vascular rejection episodes in renal transplant recipients. Lancet 1:989- 990, 1984.

54. Jacobs AD, Levenson JE, Goldie DW: Induction of acute corneal allograft rejection by alpha-2 interferon. Am J Med 82:181-182, 1987.

55. Ornellas de Souza MH, Abdelhay E, Silva MLM, et al: Late marrow allograft rejection following alpha-interferon therapy for hepatitis in a patient with paroxysmal nocturnal hemoglobinuria. Bone Marrow Transplant 9:495-497, 1992.

56. Cullis JO, Jiang YZ, Schwarer AP, et al: Donor leukocyte infusions for chronic myeloid leukemia in relapse after allogeneic bone marrow transplantation. Blood 79:1379-1380, 1992.

57. Ratanatharathorn V, Karanes C, Uberti J, et al: Phase I study of alpha-interferon augmentation of cyclosporine-induced graft vs host disease in recipients of autologous bone marrow transplantation. In press.

58. Jones RJ, Vogelsang GB, Hess AD, et al: Induction of graft- ver-

sus-host disease after autologous bone marrow transplantation. Lancet 1:754-757, 1989.

59. Carella AM, Gaozza E, Congiu A, et al: Cyclosporine-induced graft-versus-host disease after autologous bone marrow transplantation in hematological malignancies. Ann Hematol 62:156-159, 1991.

60. Hess AD, Horwitz L, Beschorner WE, et al: Development of graft-vs.-host disease-like syndrome in cyclosporine-treated rats after syngeneic bone marrow transplantation. I. Development of cytotoxic T lymphocytes with apparent polyclonal anti-Ia specificity, including autoreactivity. J Exp Med 161:718-730, 1985.

61. Geller RB, Eja AH, Beschorner WE, et al: Successful in vitro graft versus tumor effect against an Ia-bearing tumor using cyclosporine induced syngeneic graft vs host disease in the rat. Blood 74:1165, 1989.

62. Noga SJ, Horwitz L, Kim H, et al: Interferon-γ potentiates the antitumor effect of cyclosporine-induced autoimmunity. J Hematotherapy 1:75-84, 1992.

63. Schneider LC, Antin JH, Weinstein H, et al: Lymphokine profile in bone marrow transplant recipients. Blood 78:3076-3080, 1991.

64. Carlo Stella C, Cazzola M, Ganser A, et al: Recombinant gamma-interferon induces in vitro monocytic differentiation of blast cells from patients with acute nonlymphocytic leukemia and-myelodysplastic syndromes. Leukemia 2:55-59, 1988.

65. Kurzrock R, Talpaz M, Kantarjian H, et al: Therapy of chronic myelogenous leukemia with recombinant interferon-γ. Blood 70:943-947, 1987.

66. Russo D, Fanin R, Zuffa E, et al: Treatment of Ph+ chronic myeloid leukemia by gamma interferon. Blut 59:15-20, 1989.

67. Blaise D, Baume D, Olive D, et al: Association of gamma interferon and recombinant IL2 after autologous BMT. J Interferon Res 11(Suppl 1):S232, 1991.

68. Caux C, Moreau I, Saeland S, et al: Interferon-γ enhances factor-dependent myeloid proliferation of human CD34+ hematopoietic progenitor cells. Blood 79:2628-2635, 1992.

69. Jaffe HA, Buhl R, Mastrangeli A, et al: Organ specific cytokine therapy. Local activation of mononuclear phagocytes by delivery of an aerosol of recombinant interferon-γ to the human lung. J Clin Invest 88:297-302, 1991.

Chapter 8

Vaccination Strategies with Tumor Antigen in Patients with Lymphoma Undergoing Bone Marrow Transplantation

Larry W. Kwak, M.D., Ph.D.

High-dose chemo-radiotherapy followed by reconstitution with autologous bone marrow (BM) has shown considerable promise as a potentially curable approach to the therapy of lymphomas that are otherwise refractory to conventional therapeutic modalities. However, despite advances in supportive care, purging techniques, and continuing refinement of chemo-radiotherapy conditioning regimens, persistence of the underlying malignancy remains a major problem. For this reason, potential strategies for post-bone marrow transplantation (BMT) immunomodulation, and particularly, strategies aimed at enhancing a graft antilymphoma reaction would be desirable. To this end, activation of the immune system of the tumor-bearing host in a tumor-specific manner would be a worthwhile goal.

The idiotype of the surface immunoglobulin (Ig) expressed by a B-cell malignancy can serve as a tumor-specific marker, distin-

From: Spitzer T, Mazumder A: Immunotherapy and Bone Marrow Transplantation. Armonk, NY, Futura Publishing Co., Inc., © 1995.

guishing tumor cells derived from the malignant clone from other nonmalignant B cells.[1] The results in a number of experimental models have demonstrated that active immunization with tumor-derived surface Ig induces an immunoprotective effect against subsequent tumor challenge, as well as a direct antitumor effect against established tumors.[2-14] Building on these results, we immunized nine patients with B-cell lymphoma with the Ig protein derived from their own tumors after they had been treated with chemotherapy and their tumors were in remission.[15] Each received a series of subcutaneous injections of autologous Ig protein which had been conjugated to a carrier (keyhole limpet hemocyanin [KLH]), and mixed with an immunological adjuvant. In seven of the nine patients, the injections induced: sustained idiotype-specific immunological responses of the humoral type in two of the patients; the cell-mediated type in four of the patients; and both in one patient. The use of an adjuvant was essential for these immune responses. The induced antibodies bound specifically to autologous Ig idiotype, inhibited the binding of murine monoclonal anti-idiotype antibodies, and bound autologous tumor cells. Cell-mediated responses were demonstrated by the specific proliferation of immune peripheral blood mononuclear cells to the soluble Ig idiotype protein in vitro. Two patients had minimal residual measurable disease which regressed completely following the vaccination treatment. Toxicity associated with the vaccine was minimal and consisted primarily of local reactions at the injection sites. These results demonstrated that autologous Ig idiotype can be formulated into an immunogenic, tumor-specific antigen in humans with B-cell lymphoma.

Strategy for Autologous Bone Marrow Transplantation Combined with Immunoglobulin Immunization

The successful application of Ig immunization in combination with autologous BMT may depend largely on immune recovery of the host posttransplantation. Alternatively, if antitumor immunity were established before autologous BMT, this immunity would need to persist through the marrow ablative regimen to be effective in the posttransplantation period. We have explored both strategies in the preclinical model system of 38C13, a B-cell lymphoma of C3H origin. Inoculation of 1000 38C13 tumor cells intraperitoneally (I.P.) into syngeneic C3H/HeN mice results in progressive tumor growth and median survival of approximately 21 days. Single subcutaneous preimmunization with 50 mcg tumor-derived Ig coupled to KLH and emulsified in the SAF-1 adjuvant reproducibly results in approximately 60% to 80% protection from lethal tumor challenge.

We first sought to determine the efficacy of Ig vaccination in the posttransplant setting. Initial experiments suggested that mice prepared with lethal dose total body irradiation (TBI) and reconstituted with syngeneic marrow recover immune competence relatively soon after BMT. Mice prepared in this manner recovered the ability to make a primary antibody response to the KLH carrier protein as early as 3 weeks post-BMT. Guided by this observation, we tested the protective effect of Ig immunization against a subsequent lethal tumor challenge at 3 and 5 weeks post-BMT.[16] Approximately 50 C3H/HeN mice irradiated with 950 R TBI and reconstituted with BM from normal syngeneic donors were randomly assigned to five groups of approximately 10 mice each. Mice in the various groups received subcutaneous immunizations with 38C13 Ig-KLH (or with control IgM-KLH) in SAF-1 adjuvant at 3 weeks, at 5 weeks, or at both 3 and 5 weeks post-BMT. The data from this experiment are presented in Figure 1. Transplanted mice that had been immunized with 38C13 Ig-KLH at 3 weeks survived significantly longer than control animals that had been immunized with control IgM-KLH. Transplanted mice specifically immunized against tumor idiotype at 5 weeks also demonstrated significant immunoprotection after tumor challenge compared with controls. Specific immunization at this timepoint resulted in a significant number of long-term survivors, not seen with specific immunization at the earlier timepoint. This latter degree of protection was comparable with that observed in nontransplanted immunized mice. Thus, the potential for immunoprotection was fully restored by 5 weeks post-BMT. As shown in Figure 1, two serial immunizations at 3 and 5 weeks did not confer any additional immunoprotection over a single specific immunization at 5 weeks. In addition, concurrent in vitro correlates of antitumor immunity demonstrated that as early as 3 weeks post-BMT, primary antibody responses directed against the idiotype of the tumor were detectable, and the anti-idiotypic humoral response generated at 3 weeks post-BMT could be boosted by a second immunization at the 5 week timepoint.

Most studies of functional recovery of the immune system after syngeneic BMT using lethal dose TBI would have predicted that transplant-related immune depression would have been prohibitive with regard to active immunization against a tumor antigen in this early posttransplant period.[17-20] However, the unequivocal protec-

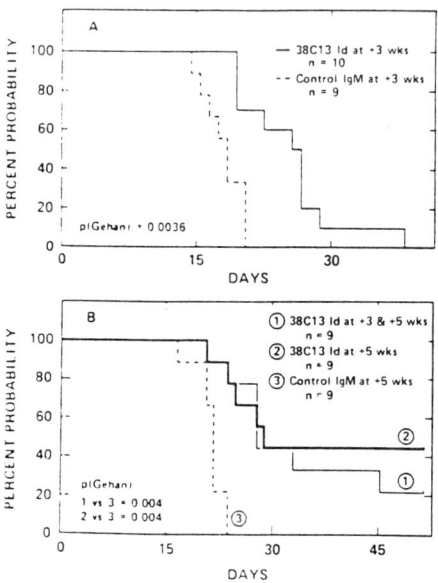

Figure 1. A: Survival of C3H/HeN mice given a single immunization with 38C13 Ig-KLH/SAF-1 or control IgM-KLH/SAF-1 3 weeks after 950 R TBI and reconstitution with syngeneic BM. Mice were injected with 1000 38C13 tumor cells I.P. at 5 weeks post-BMT. Survival (percent probability) was recorded in days post tumor challenge. B: Survival of C3H/HeN mice given single immunizations with 38C13 Ig-KLH/SAF-1 or control IgM-KLH/SAF- 1 at 5 weeks, or a combination of specific immunizations at 3 and 5 weeks, following 950 R TBI and reconstitution with syngeneic BM. All three groups of mice were injected I.P. with 1000 38C13 tumor cells from the same preparation of tumor at 7 weeks post-BMT. Reproduced with permission from Kwak, et al.[16]

tive effect of immunization against tumor-derived Ig as early as 3 and 5 weeks posttransplant indicates that the relevant immune effector mechanisms for protection against a tumor challenge were already intact at this early timepoint. Furthermore, other investigators have been able to successfully induce resistance to the L1210 leukemia by tumor immunization following lethal irradiation and syngeneic BM grafting as early as 2 to 5 weeks post-BMT.[21]

One approach to circumvent the potential obstacle of post-BMT immune depression would be to immunize the host prior to lethal dose TBI and syngeneic marrow reconstitution. Such an approach would be dependent on the establishment of antitumor immunity that would persist through the conditioning regimen. The experiment in Figure 2 was performed to test this hypothesis.[16] Approximately 30 mice were randomly assigned to receive a single immu-

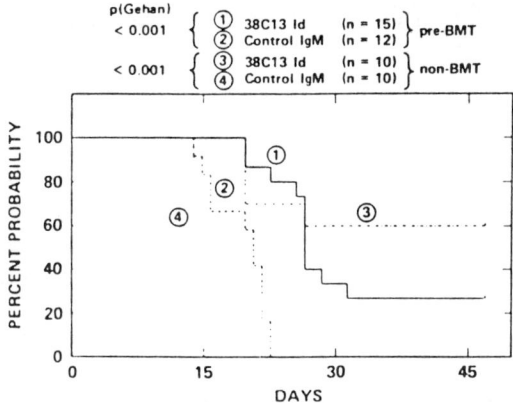

Figure 2. Survival of C3H/HeN mice given a single immunization with 38C13 Ig-KLH/SAF-1 or control IgM-KLH/SAF-1 and either transplanted or not further manipulated 2 weeks later. All mice were challenged I.P. with 1000 38C13 cells from the same preparation of tumor after 3 weeks recuperation from syngeneic BMT. Reproduced with permission from Kwak, et al.[16]

nization with 38C13 Ig-KLH or control IgM-KLH in SAF-1. Two weeks later, all mice received 950 R TBI and syngeneic marrow reconstitution; 3 weeks post-BMT, both groups were challenged with a lethal dose of tumor. Lethally irradiated and syngeneic marrow reconstituted mice that had been specifically immunized demonstrated significantly prolonged survival compared with their controls. In addition, specific immunization pre-BMT protected a significant proportion of mice (30%), which was not significantly different from the immunoprotective effect of specific immunization in nontransplanted mice.

Furthermore, determinations of serum anti-idiotypic antibody in serial serum samples from immunized transplanted mice demonstrated that in each animal, significant levels of anti-idiotypic antibody were found post-BMT at the time of tumor challenge. In fact, a direct comparison of these pre- and post-BMT antibody levels showed that in nearly all of the animals, post-BMT antibody levels were actually higher than those obtained immediately pre-BMT. Thus, the immunoprotective effect of a single Ig immunization pre-BMT was not significantly compromised by TBI. It is important to note that the conditioning regimen used in these experiments (950 R TBI) was truly BM stem cell ablative, as has been shown by other investigators.[17,19]

There are a number of examples of persistence of host immunity through BMT in humans. For example, persistence of host isohemagglutinin in ABO-incompatible marrow graft recipients has been demonstrated for up to 4 months post-BMT,[22] and in another study, antibodies against multiple viral or bacterial antigens did not show any reduction after autologous BMT when compared with pre-transplant levels.[23] In addition, recipients successfully immunized with tetanus toxoid 1 week pre-BMT showed persistence of the antibody response following TBI.[24] Another possible explanation for these results is that the anti-idiotypic immunity detected post-BMT may be derived from repopulating syngeneic donor cells stimulated by antigens still present in the recipient. However, the kinetics of the anti-idiotypic humoral response was more consistent with that of an ongoing established immune response.

In an attempt to model more closely the setting of human cancer in a tumor-bearing patient, we performed a series of experiments combining syngeneic BMT with Ig vaccination in tumor-bearing animals. In the setting of established tumor, the power of this combined therapy is also evident. In the first of such experiments shown in Figure 3A, 10^4 38C13 tumor cells were implanted subcutaneously (s.c.) in 24 mice, which were then randomized to immunization with 38C-Ig-KLH or control IgM-KLH in adjuvant. Three weekly immunizations were given to each animal, beginning on day 0. Animals in both groups received 100 mg/kg cyclophosphamide (CY) I.P. on day 10, and then 950 R TBI plus reconstitution with syngeneic BM on day 18. Both groups were monitored for tumor incidence. Clearly, the therapeutic effect of specific immunization is seen already by the time of CY administration, following which all animals in the specifically immunized group experienced complete regression of their subcutaneous tumors. Eventually, however, approximately 25% of these mice relapsed. In the experiment shown in Figure 3B, mice were again implanted with 10^4 38C13 cells s.c. and randomly assigned to either specific immunization with 38C-Ig-KLH or control IgM-KLH in adjuvant; but here treatment with immunization was not initiated until day 9, at which time almost 100% of the animals had 1 cm clearly visible subcutaneous tumors. All animals received 100 mg/kg CY I.P. as cytoreductive therapy on days 9 and 16, and then 950 R TBI plus reconstitution with syngeneic BM on day 23. Specific or nonspecific immunization was administered on days 9, 12, 18, and 27, as indicated. Again, mice were monitored for incidence of subcutaneous tumors. The therapeutic effect of specific immunization and BMT against a 1 cm macroscopically established subcutaneous tumor is less evident than when therapy is started on day 0, but a difference of approximately 40% between the experimental and control groups has been consistently observed over several experiments.

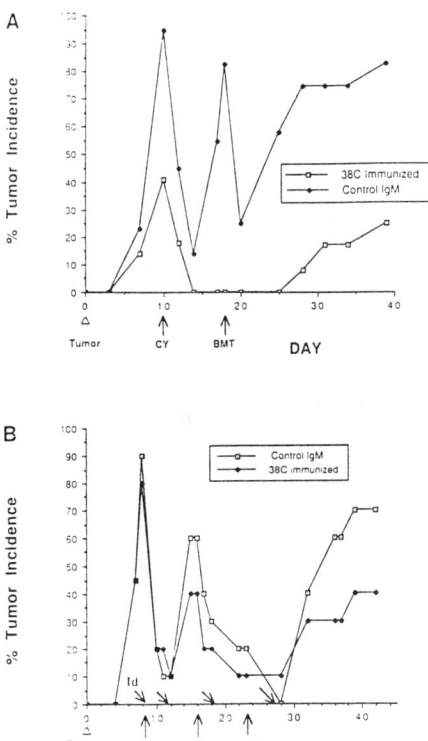

Figure 3. Therapeutic efficacy of Ig immunization combined with cyclophosphamide and BMT in tumor-bearing mice. A: Ig immunization initiated on day 0. B: Ig immunization initiated on day 9.

Thus, the therapeutic efficacy of combined pre- and post-BMT immunization has been established in the setting of a tumor-bearing host.

Immune Marrow as a Potential Anti-Tumor Element

The transfer of induced antigen-specific immunity to viral and other clinically important antigens from immune donors to BMT recipients has been explored as a potential therapeutic approach to the problem of increased host susceptibility to infection following BMT. Humoral immunity to certain antigens has been transferred from the marrow donor to the recipient in both animals and humans.[25-31]

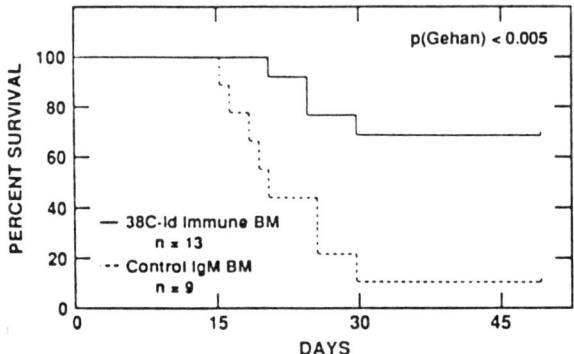

Figure 4. Survival of lethally irradiated recipients of immune (38C-Ig immune BM) or nonspecifically immune (control IgM BM) syngeneic marrow pooled from twice-immunized donors following I.P. challenge with a single preparation of 38C13 tumor cells. Reproduced with permission from Kwak, et al.[33]

The transfer of varicella zoster virus-specific cellular immunity from immune marrow donors has also been demonstrated, but only when the recipients were also immune.[32] However, to our knowledge, the transfer of antigen-specific antitumor immunity with immune marrow has not been previously studied, in large part due to the lack of a well-defined, tumor-specific antigen on most human tumors. We have used the 38C13 model to explore the ability to transfer tumor idiotype-specific immunity with BM obtained from specifically immunized donors.[33] In the experiments shown in Figure 4, syngeneic mice serving as marrow donors were immunized with either 38C13-Ig-KLH or control IgM-KLH in adjuvant, and boosted with the respective immunogen 2 weeks later. One week following this booster immunization, marrow pooled from immune or nonspecifically immune donors was used to reconstitute lethally irradiated recipients. After 3 weeks recuperation, these recipients of immune or nonspecifically immune marrow were challenged with 1000 38C13 tumor cells I.P. and monitored for survival. Recipients of immune marrow demonstrated significantly prolonged survival after tumor challenge (70% long-term survivors) compared with recipients of nonspecifically immune marrow. This full protective immunity against the 38C13 tumor was also associated with low levels of anti-idiotypic antibody in the serum of recipients of specifically immune marrow.[33]

The protective effect of immune marrow was also demonstrable in recipients which had themselves been immunized. In the experiment shown in Figure 5, normal syngeneic marrow donors were im-

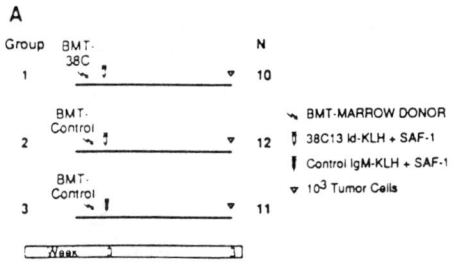

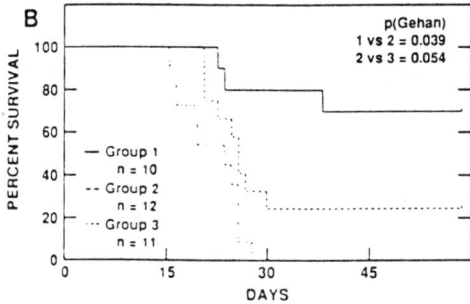

Figure 5. A: Schema for an experiment testing combined donor and recipient Ig immunization. Lethally irradiated recipients were reconstituted with marrow pooled from syngeneic donors that had been twice immunized specifically (BMT-38C) or nonspecifically (BMT-control), as described. Recipients then received a single specific or nonspecific immunization on the day of BMT as indicated. B: Survival of the three groups of mice following I.P. challenge with a single preparation of 38C13 tumor cells. Comparison of groups 2 versus 3 demonstrates the partial immunoprotective effect of specific immunization of the recipient alone. Reproduced with permission from Kwak, et al.[33]

munized twice with 38C13-Ig-KLH or control IgM-KLH in adjuvant as described above. One week following the second immunization, marrow was pooled from these immune or nonspecifically immune donors and used to reconstitute lethally irradiated syngeneic recipients. Recipients of immune marrow in this experiment also received a single subcutaneous immunization with 38C13-Ig-KLH in adjuvant on the day of transplantation; recipients of nonspecifically immune marrow were randomly assigned to receive a single immunization with either specific or control protein on the day of transplantation (Figure 5A). After 3 weeks recuperation, the resultant three groups of mice were challenged I.P. with 1000 38C13 tumor cells and monitored for survival. The tumor challenge was uniformally lethal in control nonimmune recipients of nonimmune marrow, and specific immunization of recipients of nonimmune marrow was associated with a significant prolongation of survival as well as 25% long-term survivors (group 2). The enhanced tumor resistance in group 2, compared with group 3, confirmed and extended our previous results above showing the protective effect of Ig immunization in the early posttransplant period. Of primary interest, specifically immunized recipients of immune marrow (group 1) demonstrated superior survival compared with the other two groups (70% long- term survivors). Thus, the independent immunoprotective effect of immune marrow could be demonstrated, even in lethally irradiated recipients that had been afforded an increased level of protection by Ig immunization alone posttransplantation.

In a second experiment, BM from singly immunized donors (specific versus control IgM-KLH in adjuvant) was used to reconstitute lethally irradiated recipients which were also specifically immunized with 38C13-Ig-KLH in adjuvant on the day of transplantation. After 3 weeks of recovery, both groups of mice were challenged with 1000 viable 38C13 cells and monitored for survival. As shown in Figure 6, the unequivocal protective effect of immune marrow in the setting of combined donor and recipient immunization was again demonstrated (89% long-term survivors).[fr6]

Thus, the experiments presented here clearly demonstrate that specific antitumor immunity can be transferred to lethally irradiated mice with syngeneic BM. Sufficient immunization of marrow

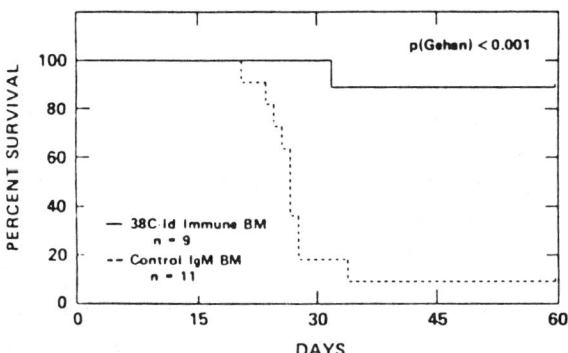

Figure 6. Combined donor and recipient Ig immunization using singly immunized syngeneic donors. Lethally irradiated recipients were reconstituted with either immune or nonspecifically immune marrow. Both groups of recipients then received a single specific immunization on the day of BMT. Shown is the survival of both groups following I.P. challenge with a single preparation of 38C13 tumor cells. Reproduced with permission from Kwak, et al.[33]

donors with purified Ig protein from 38C13 tumor was associated with the successful transfer of both protective as well as serologic anti-idiotypic immunity to the tumor. These observations are in principal directly applicable to Ig immunization of the syngeneic marrow donor of an identical twin BMT. A report of successful transfer of anti-KLH immunity from a KLH immunized marrow donor to her identical twin recipient with leukemia supports this idea,[29] although recent studies in human BMT have suggested that the expression of donor-derived antigen-specific immunity requires both an immune donor and recipient.[24,32]

Early Attempts at Post-Autologous Bone Marrow Transplantation Immunoglobulin Vaccination in Patients with Lymphoma

Two of the nine patients reported in our Phase I study[15] were patients with B-cell lymphoma in remission following autologous BMT who were vaccinated with autologous Ig-KLH plus adjuvant. The first patient was a 56 year-old man with follicular large-cell lymphoma who had received conditioning with fractionated TBI and high-dose CY 12 months prior to receiving serial Ig-KLH immunizations. The second patient was a 43 year-old female with follicular small cleaved cell lymphoma who had been prepared with [131]Iodine-anti-CD20 monoclonal antibody 32 months prior to receiving serial Ig immunizations. Both patients had recovered immunocompetence following BMT, as evidenced by the induction of both humoral and cellular responses to the carrier protein KLH. Of primary interest, both patients demonstrated T cell proliferative responses to autologous idiotype protein as well.

Strategy and Future Directions

We have demonstrated that autologous Ig idiotype can be formulated into an immunogenic, tumor-specific antigen in humans with B-cell lymphoma. The principal established by our Phase I clinical trial observations, taken together with the results of preclinical experiments in the 38C13 model, now provide a rationale for Ig immunization combined with human BMT for lymphoma. Figure 7 outlines the proposed strategy for such an approach, combining the elements of both pre- and post-BMT Ig immunization of the host. The

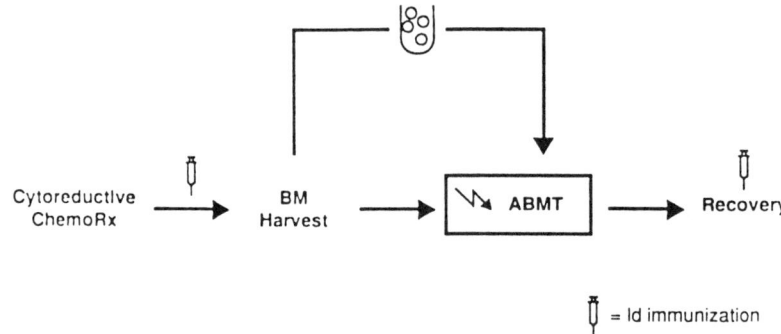

Figure 7. Strategy for autologous BMT combined with active specific immunotherapy against lymphomas. Ig immunization before marrow harvest may generate immune marrow used to reconstitute the host after high-dose chemoradiotherapy. Post-BMT Ig immunization complements this approach. Reproduced with permission from Kwak, et al.[33]

application of the immune marrow as a transfer element to autologous BMT could be accomplished by pre-BMT Ig immunization before BM harvest. If successful pre-BMT immunization of the host is accomplished, immune marrow used to reconstitute the patient after host conditioning would be spared the immunosuppressive effects of high-dose chemo-radiotherapy. An inherent assumption is that specific immunity would be preserved throughout ex vivo marrow purging and cryopreservation.

Despite the promising results of successful early posttransplant immunization in the animal model, the major concern underlying active-specific immunotherapy in the post-BMT setting remains transplant-related immune depression. Whether immune depression postautologous BMT poses an obstacle to Ig immunization in humans remains to be determined. The selection of conditioning regimens which are relatively less immunosuppressive may be an important consideration. The use of cytokines and growth factors accelerating immunological recovery post-BMT may also impact favorably in making this approach feasible. Alternatively, the ability to administer one or more carefully timed pre-BMT Ig immunizations may be crucial to the success of this approach. Our conclusion from the preclinical data presented is that a major component of antitumor immunity, if successfully established in the recipient before conditioning, does persist post-BMT. Finally, other malignancies of mature B cells, most notably multiple myeloma, may be amenable to a combined approach of BMT cytoreduction and Ig vaccination if the potential obstacles can be overcome.

References

1. Stevenson GT, Stevenson FK: Antibody to molecularly-defined antigen confined to a tumor cell surface. Nature 254:714-716, 1975.
2. Sirisinha S, Eisen HN: Autoimmune-like antibodies to the ligand-binding sites of myeloma proteins. Proc Natl Acad Sci U S A 68:3130-3135, 1971.
3. Jorgensen T, Gaudernack G, Hannestad K: Immunization with the light chain and the V_L domain of the isologous myeloma protein 315 inhibits growth of mouse plasmacytoma MOPC315. Scand J Immunol 11:29-35, 1980.
4. Daley MJ, Gebel HM, Lynch RG: Idiotype-specific transplantation resistance to MOPC-315: Abrogation by post-immunization thymectomy. J Immunol 120:1620-1624, 1978.
5. Bridges SH: Participation of the humoral immune system in the myeloma-specific transplantation resistance. J Immunol 121:479-483, 1978.
6. Freedman PM, Autry JR, Tokuda S, et al: Tumor immunity induced by preimmunization with BALB/c mouse myeloma protein. J Natl Cancer Inst 56:735-740, 1976.
7. Sugai S, Palmer DW, Talal N, et al: Protective and cellular immune responses to idiotypic determinants on cells from a spontaneous lymphoma of NZB-NZW F1 mice. J Exp Med 140:1547-1558, 1974.
8. Stevenson FK, Gordon J: Immunization with idiotypic immunoglobulin protects against development of B lymphocytic leukemia, but emerging tumor cells can evade antibody attack by modulation. J Immunol 130:970-973, 1983.
9. George AJT, Tutt AL, Stevenson FK: Anti-idiotypic mechanisms involved in the suppression of a mouse B cell lymphoma, BCL_1. J Immunol 138:628-634, 1987.
10. Kaminski MS, Kitamura K, Maloney DG, et al: Idiotype vaccination against murine B cell lymphoma: Inhibition of tumor immunity by free idiotype protein. J Immunol 138:1289-1296, 1987.
11. Campbell MJ, Carroll W, Kon S, et al: Idiotype vaccination against murine B cell lymphoma: Humoral and cellular responses elicited by tumor-derived immunoglobulin M and its molecular subunits. J Immunol 139:2825-2833, 1987.
12. Campbell MJ, Esserman L, Byars NE, et al: Idiotype vaccination against murine B cell lymphoma: Humoral and cellular requirements for the full expression of antitumor immunity. J Immunol 145:1029-1036, 1990.

13. George AJT, Folkard SG, Hamblin TJ, et al: Idiotypic vaccination as a treatment for a B cell lymphoma. J Immunol 141:2168-2174, 1988.
14. Campbell MJ, Esserman L, Levy R: Immunotherapy of established murine B cell lymphoma: Combination of idiotype immunization and cyclophosphamide. J Immunol 141:3227-3233, 1988.
15. Kwak LW, Campbell MJ, Czerwinski DK, et al: Induction of immune responses in patients with B-cell lymphoma against the surface-immunoglobulin idiotype expressed by their tumors. N Engl J Med 327:1209-1215, 1992.
16. Kwak LW, Campbell MJ, Zelenetz AD, et al: Combined syngeneic bone marrow transplantation and immunotherapy of a murine B-cell lymphoma: Active immunization with tumor-derived idiotypic immunoglobulin. Blood 76:2411-2417, 1990.
17. Samlowski WE, Crump CL: Recovery of contact hypersensitivity responses following murine bone marrow transplantation: Comparison of gamma-irradiation and busulfan as preparative marrow ablative agents. Blood 70:1910, 1987.
18. Samlowski WE, Araneo BA, Butler MO, et al: Peripheral lymph node helper T-cell recovery after syngeneic bone marrow transplantation in mice prepared with either γ-irradiation or busulfan. Blood 74:1436, 1989.
19. Merluzzi VJ, Welte K, Last-Barney K, et al: Production and response to interleukin 2 in vitro and in vivo after bone marrow transplantation in mice. J Immunol 134:2426, 1985.
20. Merluzzi VJ, Savage DM, Smith MD, et al: Lymphokine-activated killer cells are generated before classical cytotoxic T lymphocytes after bone marrow transplantation in mice. J Immunol 135:1702, 1985.
21. Skorski T, Kawalec M: Recovery of the ability to induce immune resistance against L1210 lymphatic leukemia in semisyngeneic 2F1 mice after lethal irradiation and reconstitution with bone marrow purged of leukemia with mafosfamide (ASTA Z 7654). Bone Marrow Transplant 2:435, 1987.
22. Witherspoon RP, Storb R, Ochs HD, et al: Recovery of antibody production in human allogeneic marrow graft recipients: Influence of time post-transplantation, the presence or absence of chronic graft-versus-host disease, and antithymocyte globulin treatment. Blood 58:360, 1981.
23. Gorin NC, Muller JY, Solmon C, et al: Immunocompetence following autologous bone marrow transplantation. Exp Hematol 7:327, 1979.

24. Wimperis JZ, Prentice HG, Karayiannis P, et al: Transfer of a functioning humoral immune system in transplantation of T-lymphocyte-depleted bone marrow. Lancet 1:339, 1986.
25. Stoner RD, Bond VP: Antibody formation by transplanted bone marrow, spleen, lymph nodes and thymus cells in irradiated recipients. J Immunol 91:185, 1963.
26. Gengozian N, Makinodan T, Shekarchi IC: Transplantation of antibody-forming cells in lethally irradiated mice. J Immunol 86:113, 1961.
27. Garver RM, Santos GW, Cole LJ: Specific hemagglutinins in x-irradiated, bone marrow treated mice following differential immunization of host and donor. J Immunol 83:57, 1959.
28. Gross-Wilde H, Krumbacher K, Schuning F, et al: Immune transfer studies in canine allogeneic marrow graft donor-recipient pairs. Transplantation 42:64, 1986.
29. Starling KA, Falletta JM, Fernbach DJ: Immunologic chimerism as evidence of bone marrow graft acceptance in an identical twin with acute lymphocytic leukemia. Exp Hematol 3:244, 1975.
30. Lum LG, Munn NA, Schanfield MS, et al: The detection of specific antibody formation to recall antigens after human bone marrow transplantation. Blood 67:582, 1986.
31. Lum LG, Seigneuret MC, Storb R: The transfer of antigen-specific humoral immunity from marrow donors to marrow recipients. J Clin Immunol 6:389, 1986.
32. Kato S, Yabe H, Yabe M, et al: Studies on transfer of varicella-zoster-virus specific T-cell immunity from bone marrow donor to recipient. Blood 75:806, 1990.
33. Kwak LW, Campbell MJ, Zelenetz AD, et al: Transfer of specific immunity to B-cell lymphoma with syngeneic bone marrow in mice: A strategy for using autologous marrow as an anti-tumor therapy. Blood 78:2768-2772, 1991.

Chapter 9

Capillary Leak Syndrome After Bone Marrow Transplantation:
Potential Impact on the Toxicities of Immunotherapy In These Patients

Richard Cahill, M.D.

Given the persistent problem of disease relapse despite having reached maximum doses of chemotherapy and irradiation in the preparative regimens for bone marrow transplantation (BMT), additional therapy for some malignancies will be required. Therefore, the role of cytokines and other biological response modifiers following transplantation will likely expand. However, there are considerable toxicities associated with the use of these therapies that may enhance some of the transplanted related toxicities that already occur. The cytokines interleukin (IL)-6, granulocyte macrophage-colony stimulating factor (GM-CSF), tumor necrosis factor (TNF)-α, interferon (IFN)-γ, and IL-1 have been implicated in most post-

From: Spitzer T, Mazumder A: Immunotherapy and Bone Marrow Transplantation. Armonk, NY, Futura Publishing Co., Inc., © 1995.

Table 1

Toxicity Associated With Interleukin-2 in Autologous and T-Cell
Depleted Allogeneic Bone Marrow Transplantation Patients

Organ	Symptoms
Systemic	Chills, fever, weight gain, rash
Respiratory	Dyspnea, interstitial edema, pleural effusions, respiratory failure
Hepatic	Hyperbilirubinemia, veno-occlusive disease
Renal	Azotemia
Cardiovascular	Hypotension
Gastrointestinal	Nausea, diarrhea
Infections	Viral, gram positive bacterial
CNS	Mental status changes
Hematopoietic	Thrombocytopenia, lymphopenia, and eosinophilia

transplant-related complications including graft-versus-host disease (GVHD) and hepatic veno-occlusive disease (VOD),[1] and are the important secondary cytokines responsible for the vascular leak syndrome during IL-2 therapy.[2-9] Thus, patients undergoing BMT may experience additional difficulty after the preparative regimen and during the posttransplant period potentially limiting the therapeutic use of these factors. IL-2 therapy after transplant has been used primarily in the autologous setting and in allogeneic patients who receive T-cell- depleted (TCD) transplants. The toxicities (Table 1) in these situations, however, have been minimal compared to IL-2 therapy in cancer patients. The concerns about posttransplant IL-2 in the non-T cell allogeneic transplant recipients include the enhancement of vascular permeability, as well as an increase in acute GVHD.

Capillary Leak Syndrome in Bone Marrow Transplantation Patients

Endothelial injury following the preparative regimen for BMT occurs in both allogeneic and autologous marrow transplant patients, but has not been well characterized. It was first reported by Powles in 1984 in mismatched donor-related transplant recipients[10] and more recently in some detail by our group.[11,12] In most respects, the clinical signs and symptoms resemble the leaky capillaries seen during IL-2 therapy but tend to be more insidious in onset and related to the presence of white blood cells during the time of engraftment. It is of note that Powles et al. were only able to prevent the syndrome by T-cell depletion[10]

Capillary leak syndrome (CLS) in BMT patients is characterized by a rash, fever, peripheral edema, and excessive weight gain (>5% to 10% of baseline or >10% to 20% of the day 0 weight). More serious manifestations include: respiratory distress, and in some cases fatal respiratory failure; secondary to pleural effusions and interstitial edema, ascites, and liver function abnormalities that are compatible with VOD (hyperbilirubinemia out of proportion to elevated transaminases); confusion and/or convulsions; and azotemia or renal failure. During IL-2 therapy, cancer patients experience a similar, but more acute, clinical picture which resolves following discontinuation of the IL-2 injections.

Incidence and mortality of CLS in our series were observed to be more apparent in the allogeneic setting. Other predisposing factors included previous antineoplastic therapy, interval from diagnosis, and location (chest or abdomen) of radiation therapy. Lymphomas of the chest or mediastinum were more prone to develop effusions and pulmonary edema during the preparative regimen, as well as during engraftment, even if they had not had previous radiation therapy to the tumor bed. No differences in incidence of CLS were seen using busulfan/cyclophosphamide (BU/CY) or total body irradiation/cyclophosphamide (TBI/CY) as the preparative regimen. However, when escalating doses of etoposide (VP-16) were used, the syndrome was more common. In patients receiving buffy coat (BC) infusions or backup marrow infusions, the syndrome occurred acutely and involved, predominantly, the lungs. All patients who developed fungal sepsis and received Amphotericin B responded temporarily to steroids, but eventually died of respiratory failure.

Other clinical scenarios where a CLS may also occur include reperfusion injury,[13-15] transfusion related acute lung injury (TRALI),[16,17] adult respiratory distress syndrome (ARDS),[18,19] and the retinoic acid syndrome.[20]

The Pathogenesis of the Capillary Leak Syndrome in Bone Marrow Transplantation Patients and Its Similarity to Interleukin-2 Therapy

The optimal antitumor effect of IL-2 therapy most likely occurs when administered immediately after BMT,[21] but considerable apprehension exists regarding toxicities with such early administration of IL-2. The toxicity of IL-2 is dependent upon an intact immune system[9] as well as several other factors, most prominently, dose and schedule. High dose IL-2 is considered >1.5 mg/m^2 or 0.1 nmol/L. An IV bolus dose of 10 mg, equivalent to 180 million U IV, is the maximum tolerated dose and produces the same side effects as does 1 mg given over 24 hours.[9] High-dose IL-2 stimulates natural killer (NK) cells to release cytokines, which in turn cause the release of secondary cytokines from host cells, ie, IL-1, TNF-α, and GM-CSF. At low doses, however, IL-2 promotes the proliferation of a minor subset of NK cells, namely the 10% to 20% that express a high-affinity IL-2R, and which account for only 1% of peripheral blood leukocytes.

Toxicities from IL-2 in autologous and TCD allogeneic transplants, surprisingly, have been manageable, and suggest that IL-2 toxicity may have a similar relationship to T-cell activation as demonstrated by Rosenstein and Cotran in the mouse[22,23] and alluded to by Powles in BMT patients.[10] Although the clinical signs and symptoms of CLS in BMT patients and during IL-2 therapy are similar, the initiation of endothelial injury appears to be different because BMT patients receive cytoreductive conditioning therapy followed by the infusion of allogeneic or autologous bone marrow (BM).

Electron microscopy of IL-2 treated patients[24,25] and BMT patients[26] with CLS has confirmed similar changes in the capillary endothelium that allows the passage of fluid, red and white cells, and protein freely into the interstitial spaces. With light microscopy, a perivascular mononuclear cellular infiltrate (T cells, monocytes, and Langerhan's dendritic cells) characteristic of a delayed-type hypersensitivity reaction (DTH) can be seen in leprosy patients injected intradermally with IL-2.[25] The pulmonary and hepatic vasculature in mice with IL-2 toxicity reveal a marked lymphoid cell infiltration with predominantly Thy1$^+$ and asialo-GM1$^+$ cells.[27]

The toxicity of IL-2 is also mediated via soluble factors, including TNF, IFN, and IL-6.[2,7,23,28-31] Elevated levels posttransplant of TNF, IFN-γ, and IL-6 have been found in patients before the onset of GVHD and VOD.[1,32-35] Although we have been unable to confirm these data, we have found marked elevations of the two arachidonic acid metabolites, LTE4 and TxB2, in both autologous and allogeneic patients with CLS.[11] The ability of these products of the lipo-oxygenase and cyclo-oxygenase pathways to cause leaky capillaries has been confirmed in animal models,[36] as well as in animals given IL-2.[13] These products are chemotactic for white cells,[37-39] cause vasoconstriction in the renal[36,40] and pulmonary vascular bed resulting in pulmonary hypertension and edema,[41] activate white cells,[42,43] and by themselves activate the endothelium resulting in leaky capillaries.[13,41] They are also implicated in the priming of other cells to enhance the production of cytokines.[36]

The severity of CLS in our BMT patient population setting was most pronounced in the presence of leukocytes; the majority of patients (62%) experienced the syndrome during engraftment and CLS manifested itself in two patients after rapid steroid taper. In a smaller number of patients (31%), CLS occurred during, or immediately after, the preparative regimen and included two patients who received BC infusions. Pulmonary edema with or without effusions and hemorrhage improved in six of nine patients as the white cells disappeared but reappeared during engraftment. The two patients (7%) that received backup marrow had an acute onset of leaky capillaries with serious pulmonary decompensation resulting in one fatality. Brandt et al. reported an incidence of 11% CLS in autologous patients receiving recombinant human granulocyte macrophage-colony stimulating factor (rHuGM-CSF) after transplant.[44] The fluid and rash completely disappeared after stopping the CSF. A major role for activated white cells in reperfusion injury,[13-15,30] TRALI,[16,17] and retinoic acid syndrome[20] has been established. However, the occurrence of ARDS in neutropenic patients suggest that multiple mechanisms can produce leaky capillaries,[45] including activation of host cells by infectious agents and their treatment.[46]

Polymorphonuclear leukocytes (PMN) have not thus far received the attention that lymphocytes have in IL-2 therapy. There is evidence that PMNs may play a major role in the development of CLS therapy. Welbourn et al. pretreated rats prior to infusion with selective antirat neutrophil antibodies, and observed a decrease in the production of thromboxane and a preclusion of the pulmonary edema.[8] In the absence of PMNs, a major source of TNF,[31] anti-TNF antibodies,[47] or drugs like pentoxifylline fail to prevent IL-2 toxicity.[48] Recently, Meir and colleagues were able to correct the defect in white cell function with low-dose steroids, and they noted a decrease in TNF production by PMNs without losing the antitumor effect of the IL-2-stimulated cells.[49]

During IL-2 therapy there is an increased incidence of gram positive bacterial infections, particularly central venous catheter infections.[50] Several abnormalities in PMN function have been elucidated including a defect in chemotaxis,[51] and the decreased expression of an Fc receptor important for attachment of the PMN to the organisms.[52] This reported defect in white cell chemotaxis may prevent more serious toxicity from occurring by decreasing the presence of PMNs at the site of endothelial injury. However, there is also marked complement activation[6,53] and IL-6[7] production, each of which is chemotactic for white cells. Controversy continues as to whether the white cells are primed and demonstrate increased[54] or decreased superoxide production during IL-2 therapy.[52,55] In the latter case, the activated or "deactivated" cells would not be able to function properly in face of a gram positive infection, or contribute to the destruction of the endothelium.

Increased levels of TNF and IFN have been found in both animal models and human recipients after IL-2 therapy, and have been shown to be initially responsible for the toxicity.[2,23,27,28,30,47,49,57] These cytokines activate the endothelium and cause the expression of Class I and Class II antigens.[56] IFN-γ is thought to be primarily responsible for migration of lymphokine-activated killer (LAK) cells across the endothelium[58] and is dependent upon the adhesion molecule lymphocyte function-associated antigen (LFA)-1. It is also partly responsible for the decrease in red cell and platelet production.[59] If the animal is pretreated with anti-TNF antibodies, CLS develops, which can be explained either by the direct action of NK cells[60] on the endothelium or the recruitment of T cells capable of adhesion and lysis.[9,61] Conversely, in NK-depleted mice continuous infusion of IL-2 ultimately results in the syndrome, suggesting that other host cells (eg, pulmonary macrophages) or regenerating NK cells may become activated and produce cytokines and other mediators capable of causing the CLS syndrome.[27]

The effect of IL-2 on lymphocytes may well be critical to the severity of the toxicity after allogeneic BMT. Early after the initiation of IL-2 therapy, patients experience a fall in the lymphocyte count followed by a lymphocytosis immediately after stopping therapy. This indicates that the lymphopenia is due either to margination, or the adhesion of lymphocytes to the endothelium.[9,59,62] Following BMT, patients have a severe deficit in T-cell function, in addition to the small numbers of cluster designation (CD)4+ and CD5+ lymphocytes and NK cells.[55] Production of mitogen or antigen stimulated IL-2, TNF, or IFN is markedly diminished. The cell repertoire in experimental animals and patients receiving IL-2, however, is somewhat controversial. Patients receiving chronic doses of IL-2 show a transient lymphopenia followed by an increase in NK and LAK cells bearing the Leu-19+ marker which are either CD16+ or CD16-.[63,64,69] Urba and Higuchi also found an increase in the expression of CD38 and CD8 antigens, whereas McMannis et al. found a decrease in the percentage of CD8+ cells. Mice experience a lymphopenia in the first 24 hours with a decrease in CD4+ cells and an increase in splenic CD3+CD4-CD8- cells at 3 and 4 days.[64,65] It was later established that high-dose IL-2 inhibited CD4+ activity but had no effect on CD8[65] cells responsible for the graft-versus-leukemia (GVL) effect.[65] It is of note that CD8[+] T-LAK cells also migrate more vigorously than CD4[+] T-LAK cells.[57] Gately et al. analyzed the body fluids and pulmonary vasculature and found high numbers of Thy1[+] and asialo-GM1[+] cells as well a substantial number of Lyt-2[+] cells.[27] With low-dose IL-2 infusions, the toxicity as well as the antitumor effect are less and these patients have a lymphocytosis composed mainly of NK cells (CD3[-],CD56[+]).[66] In an animal model, the addition of IL-2-treated BM along with low-dose IL-2 posttransplant has increased the number of NK cells as well as the efficacy of the treatment without increasing toxicity.[21]

Experience in the Literature Using Interleukin-2 in Bone Marrow Transplantation Patients

Major toxicity has, for the most part, occurred only at high doses in autologous BMT patients[67-74] and TCD allogeneic BMT patients,[71] or when LAK cells were given.[75] Very few deaths have been reported and those deaths were associated with other complications. Weisdorf et al., in their series of 14 patients who received a dose of 2.0×10^6 U/m^2 per day, reported 4 deaths; 2 with pulmonary edema, 1 with a viral infection, and 1 with pancytopenia.[68] One autologous patient died of pulmonary edema in Hamon's series of seven patients.[72] Three reports of significant thrombocytopenia in patients treated with IL-2 at doses of 3.0×10^6 U/m^2 per day,[69,70] or LAK cells[75] are of concern. Negrier et al. reported a delay in BM recovery which they attributed to the toxic effects of carmustine (BCNU) in the preparative regimen[71] Although IL-2 stimulates IFN production, recovery of BM in these patients has, for the most part, been accelerated.[68]

Hypotension has been a common occurrence in the IL-2-treated BMT patients, but no significant cardiotoxicity has been reported with the exception of one patient who also received IFN.[73] High fevers (>39$dgC) accompanied by chills and rigors have been an important problem requiring acetaminophen and nonsteroidal antiinflamatory agents.

Potential problems that have not been reported in the autologous or TCD allogeneic patients, but may occur in the non-TCD allografts is an increase in GVHD. The purpose of the therapy is to increase the graft-versus-tumor (GVT) effect which may also be an important component of GVHD. Mice treated with IL-2 developed accelerated lethal GVHD that could be prevented only by T-cell depletion.[74] Favrot et al. reported one child with neuroblastoma who received a non-TCD marrow transplant and developed mild GVHD that responded to discontinuation of the IL-2 and steroid therapy.[76] Although Soiffer reported an increase in CD4+ cells after low-dose IL-2, GVHD did not occurr in the autologous BMT or TCD patients.[70] In an animal model, IL-2 given in the first 3 days protects against acute GVHD, at least in part by inhibition of the CD4+ T cells that are responsible for GVHD but not GVL.[65] Duncombe et al. are concerned that IL-2-activated major histocompatibility complex (MHC) unrestricted killer cells that attack normal marrow fibroblasts, as well as virally infected targets, might result in severe marrow hypoplasia in the setting of cytomegalovirus (CMV) infections.[77]

Experience with Interleukin-2-Activated Peripheral Blood Stem Cells, Autologous Bone Marrow and/or Low-Dose Interleukin-2 Infusions

In our series of 15 breast cancer patients who received peripheral blood stem cells (PBSC) cultured for 24 hours in IL-2 (n=5) or 2 weeks (n=5) of IL-2 infusions (6×10^5 I.U./m^2 per day), 1 patient experienced congestive heart failure. Eleven patients (73%) developed biopsy proven GVHD of the skin; and 5 (33%), of the gut.

Ten patients with lymphoma (n=5) and leukemia (n=5) have undergone autologous transplant with either short- or long-term culture of their marrow with IL-2. As seen in Table 2, there was considerable toxicity, expecially in the lymphoma patients with mediastinal involvement which has been previously reported in patients with IL-2. One patient (Unique Patient Number [UPN] 271) died of respiratory failure.

In seven instances, IL-2 was administered for 1 to 4 weeks after the IL-2-cultured marrow and PBSC. Three leukemia and two lymphoma patients who were given additional IL-2-cultured PBSC and low-dose IL-2 infusions developed, during the first week, high fevers, diarrhea, liver function abnormalities, and skin rashes. All biopsies of the skin and sigmoid colon were consistent with GVHD. A presumptive diagnosis of liver involvement was made with the associated gut and skin changes and the improvement after steroid therapy, as well as stopping the IL-2. One acute myeloid leukemia (AML) patient (UPN 289) died from infection and before engraft-

Table 2
Complications of Interleukin-2 Activated Bone Marrow and Stem Cells

UPN/Age	Disease	IL-2 Infusion	CLS	GVHD
280/46	NHL	No	0	0
271/28	HD	No	++++	0
292/17	HD	No	++	0
289/44	NHL	1 Week	0	0
293/55	CML	4 Weeks	++	++
317/40	AML	1 Week*	+++	++
312/31	NHL	1 Week*	+++	++
322/56	CML	2 Weeks	+	+
321/39	NHL	3 Weeks	++	+

*IL-2 infusions stopped after 1 week; UPN: unique patient number; IL: Interleukin; CLS: Capillary leak syndrome; GVHD: Graft-vs-host disease; NHL: non-Hodgkins lymphoma; HD: Hodgkins disease; CML: Chronic myeloid leukemia; AML: Acute myeloid leukemia.

ment. Experience in the literature concerning the use of IL-2 in bone marrow transplant patients suggests that it is more difficult to administer and should be delayed.[68] It is of note that our patients were also getting PBSC, or additional white cells. However, the majority of patients responded to steroids and the discontinuation of the IL-2.

Therapy: Practical and Theoretical

Many of the problems encountered during IL-2 therapy are also seen in the BMT setting. The increased capillary permeability frequently results in hypovolemia and edema.[78] This loss of intravascular fluid results in a decrease in renal blood flow and glomerular filtration. The ascites, interstitial edema, and pleural effusions further diminish pulmonary and liver function.

The cause and treatment of the hypovolemia and hypotension is controversial. Some investigators believe there is a direct effect of IL-2 on the cardiac muscle resulting in ischemia, arrhythmias and the hypotension.[4] The fluid retention is a result of the oliguria,[79] and the cardiac dysfunction is due to the hypovolemia, as suggested by several investigators.[5,78,80-82] This requires exogenous fluid administration, and attempts to reduce fluid administration have led to accelerated increases in serum creatinine and anuria.[81,82] Dopamine has been used as a vasopressor in an attempt to avoid more fluid administration.[5] Patient recovery is usually accomplished after the IL-2 infusion is terminated. Administration of corticosteroids has also been successful, but may interfere with the action of the LAK cells against the tumor.[83,84] Low dose dexamethasone, however, has been shown recently to correct the defect in chemotaxis and decrease the toxicity without interfering with the efficacy of the LAK cells.[49]

Patients with preexisting cardiac dysfunction have been excluded from consideration of BMT because of the severe cardiac toxicity of the CY-containing preparative regimen. Despite the high doses of chemo-radiotherapy administered during the pretransplant period and the known negative inotropic effect of leukotrienes on the heart,[36] cardiac dysfunction following the transplant is usually not a significant clinical problem. The intravascular depletion seen after IL-2 therapy is usually not as profound, but is typically more insidious and parallels engraftment. Renal dose dopamine ($2 \mu g/kg$ per minute) is often used as a vasodilator to overcome the pre-renal failure by maintaining adequate renal flow.[85] It may have a similar benefit in the microvascular injury of the liver. An additional advantage of dopamine is its ability to interfere with NADPH oxidase, a white blood cell enzyme responsible for superoxide formation.[86] Furosemide appears to be beneficial in maintaining an adequate blood flow to the kidney tubules due to the release of prostacyclin[87] which is reduced after irradiation.[88]

As discussed above, some patients in our series experienced CLS during the preparative regimen when the white cell count was normal; the toxicities of low-dose IL-2 administered in the first 5 days after allogeneic transplant may not be as profound, in part, because of the absence of circulating donor white cells. Problems could arise in the allogeneic patients if the IL-2 therapy is extended by continuous stimulation of donor T cells and host mononuclear cells as illustrated in mice depleted of NK cells before IL-2 therapy.[27,41,61]

Side effects of high-dose IL-2 therapy and/or LAK cells, especially fever, have been treated with multiple drugs, some of which have been implicated in other organ damage.[5] The cyclo-oxygenase inhibitor, indomethacin, has been used extensively to treat the chills and fever associated with IL-2 therapy. We have not used indomethacin in the BMT setting, due to fear that it will shift the arachidonic metabolism to the 5-lipo-oxygenase pathway and increase the production of the leukotrienes. Pulses of corticosteroids have had an immediate beneficial effect, unless they are being used for prophylaxis or treatment of severe GVHD.

References

1. Antin JH, Ferrara LM: Cytokine dyregulation and acute graft-versus-host-disease. Blood 80:2964-2968, 1992.

2. Heslop HE, Gottlieb DJ, Bianchi ACM, et al: In vivo induction of gamma interferon and tumor necrosis factor by interleukin-2 infusion following intensive chemotherapy or autologous marrow transplantation. Blood 74:1374-1378, 1989.
3. Klausner JM, Paterson IS, Mannick JA, et al: Reperfusion pulmonary edema. JAMA 261:1030-1035, 1989.
4. Hawkins MJ, Sznol M: The cardiovascular effects of human recombinant cytokines. In FM Muggia, MD Green, JL Speyer (eds): Cancer Treatment and the Heart. Baltimore, Md, John Hopkins University Press, 1992, pp 296-327.
5. Siegel JP, Puri RK: Interleukin-2 toxicity. J Clin Oncol 9:694-704, 1991.
6. Wagstaff J, Vermorker JB, Schwartsmann G, et al: A progress report of a Phase I study of interferon-γ and interleukin-2 and some comments on the mechanism of the toxicity due to interleukin-2. Cancer Treat Rev 16:105-109, 1989.
7. Musso T, Espinoza-Delgado I, Pulkki K, et al: Il-2 induces Il-6 production in human monocytes. J Immunol 148:795-800, 1992.
8. Welbourn R, Goldman G, Kobzik L, et al: Interleukin-2 induces early multisystem organ edema mediated by neutrophils. Ann Surg 214:181-186, 1991.
9. Smith KA: Lowest dose interleukin-2 immunotherapy. Blood 81:1414-1423, 1993.
10. Powles R, Pedrazzini A, Crofts M, et al: Mismatched family bone marrow transplantation. Semin Hematol 21:182-187, 1984.
11. Cahill RA, Zhao Y, Murphy RC, et al: High urinary leukotriene E4 (LTE4) and thromboxane 2 (TxB2) levels are associated with capillary leak syndrome in bone marrrow transplant patients. In B Samuelson, T Ramwell (eds): Advances in Prostaglandin, Thromboxane, and Leukotriene Research. Volume 21B. New York, NY, Raven Press, 1991, pp 525-528.
12. Cahill RA, Spitzer TR, Mazumder A, et al: Marrow engraftment and clinical manifestations of capillary leak syndrome. In press.
13. Klausner JM, Paterson IS, Morel NM, et al: Role of thromboxane in interleukin 2-induced lung injury in sheep. Cancer Res 49:3542-3549, 1989.
14. Lucchesi BR: Myocardial ischemia, reperfusion and free radical injury. Am J Cardiol 65:141-231, 1990.
15. Odeh M: The role of reperfusion-induced injury in the pathogenesis of crush syndrome. N Engl J Med 324:1417-1422, 1991.
16. Seeger W, Schneider U, Kreusler B, et al: Reproduction of transfusion-related acute lung injury in an ex vivo lung model. Blood 76:1438-1444, 1990.

17. Sillman C, Johnson C, Clay K, et al: Lipids develop during the routine storage of blood that prime neutrophils through the platelet activating factor (PAF) receptor and are structurally distinct-from PAF. Blood 80:261a, 1992.
18. Bell RC, Coalson JJ, Smith JD, et al: Multiple organ system failure and infection in adult respiratory distress syndrome. Ann Intern Med 99:293-298, 1983.
19. Tamashefski JF: Pulmonary pathology of the adult respiratory distress syndrome. Clin Chest Med 2:593-619, 1990.
20. Frankel SR, Eardley A, Lauwers G, et al: The "retinoic acid syndrome" in acute promyelocytic leukemia. Ann Intern Med 117:292-296, 1992.
21. Charak BS, Brynes RK, Katsuda S, et al: Induction of graft versus leukemia effect in bone marrow transplantation: Dosage and time schedule dependency of interleukin-2 therapy. Cancer Res 51:2015-2020, 1991.
22. Rosenstein M, Ettinghausen SE, Rosenberg SA: Extravasation of intravascular fluid mediated by the systemic administration of recombinant interleukin 2. J Immunol 137:1735-1739, 1986.
23. Cotran RS, Pober JS, Gimbrone MA, et al: Endothelial activation during interleukin 2 immunotherapy. A possible mechanism for the vascular leak syndrome. J Immunol 139:1883-1888, 1987.
24. Fujita S, Puri RK, Zu-Xi LYu, et al: An ultrastructural study of in vivo interactions between lymphocytes and endothelial cells in the pathogenesis of the vascular leak syndrome induced by interleukin-2. Cancer 68:2169-2174, 1991.
25. Kaplan G, Britton WJ, Hancock GE, et al: The systemic influence of recombinant interleukin 2 on the manifestations of lepromatous leprosy. J Exp Med 173:993-1006, 1991.
26. Cohen H, Bull HA, Seddon A, et al: Vascular endothelial cell function and ultrastructure in thrombotic microangiopathy following allogeneic bone marrow transplantation. Eur J Haematol 43:207-214, 1989.
27. Gately MK, Anderson TD, Hayes TJ: Role of asialo-gm1- positive lymphoid cells in mediating the toxic effects of recombinant Il-2 in mice. J Immunol 141:189-200, 1988.
28. Gemlo BR, Palladino MA, Jaffe HS, et al: Circulating cytokines in patients with metastatic cancer treated with recombinant interleukin 2 and lymphokine-activated killer cells. Cancer Res 48:5864-5867, 1988.
29. Ettinghausen SE, Puri RK, Rosenberg SA: Increased vascular permeability in organs mediated by the systemic administration

of lymphokine-activated killer cells and recombinant inter-leukin-2 in mice. J Natl Cancer Inst 80:177-188, 1988.

30. Pober JS, Cotran RS: Cytokines and endothelial cell biology Physiol Rev 70:427-451, 1990.
31. Wei S, Blanchard DK, Liu JH, et al: Activation of tumor necrosis factor-α production from human neutrophils by Il-2 via Il-2-Rβ. J Immunol 150:1979-1987, 1993.
32. Holler E, Kolb HJ, Moller A, et al: Increased serum levels of tumor necrosis factor α precede major complication of bone marrow transplantation. Blood 75:1011-1016, 1990.
33. Piguet P, Grau GE, Allet B, et al: Tumor necrosis factor/cachectin is an effector of skin and gut lesions of the acute phase of graft-vs-host disease. J Exp Med 166:1280-1289, 1987.
34. Symington FW, Pepe MS, Chen AB, et al: Serum tumor necrosis factor alpha associated with acute graft-versus-host-disease in humans. Transplantation 50:518-524, 1990.
35. Symington FW, Symington BE, Liu PY, et al: The relationship of serum Il-6 levels to acute graft-versus-host disease and hepatorenal disease after human bone marrow transplantation. Transplantation 54:457-462, 1992.
36. Lewis RA, Austen KF, Soberman RJ: Mechanisms of disease: Leukotrienes and other products of the 5-lipoxygenase pathway-biochemistry and relation to pathobiology in human diseases. N Engl J Med 323:645-656, 1990.
37. Buchanan MR, Vazquez MJ, Gimbrone MA: Arachidonic acid metabolism and the adhesion of human polymorphonuclear leukocytes to cultured vascular endothelial cells. Blood 62:889-895, 1983.
38. Doukas J, Shepro D, Hechtman HB: Vasoactive amines directly modify endothelial cells to affect polymorphonuclear leukocyte diapedesis in vitro. Blood 69:1563-1569, 1987.
39. Goldman G, Welbourn R, Valeri CR, Shepro D, Hechtman HB: Thromboxane A_2 induces leukotriene B_4 synthesis that in turn mediates neutrophil diapedesis via CD 18 activation. Microvasc Res 41:367-375, 1991.
40. Epstein M, Lifschitz MD: Renal eicosanoids as determinants of renal function in liver disease. Hepatology 7:1359-1367, 1987.
41. Ferro TJ, Johnson A, Everitt J, et al: Il-2 induces pulmonary edema and vasoconstriction independent of circulating lymphocytes. J Immunol 142:1916-1921, 1989.
42. Abramson DB, Leszczynska-Piziak J, Weissmann G: Arachiodonic acid as a second messenger. Interactions with a GTP-binding protein of human neutrophils. J Immunol 147:231-236, 1987.

43. Sakata A, Ida E, Tominaga M, et al: Arachidonic acid acts as an intracellular activator of NADPH-oxidase in Fc receptor- mediated superoxide generation in macrophages. J Immunol 138:4353-4359, 1987.
44. Brandt SJ, Peters WP, Atwater SK, et al: Effect of recombinant human granulocyte-macrophage colony-stimulating factor on hematopoietic reconstitution after high-dose chemotherapy and autologous bone marrow transplantation. N Engl J Med 318:869-876, 1988.
45. Ognibene FP, Martin SE, Parker MM, et al: Adult respiratory distress syndrome in patients with severe neutropenia. N Engl J Med 315:547-551, 1986.
46. Chia JK, Pollack M: Amphotericin B induces tumor necrosis factor production by murine macrophages. J Infect Dis 159:113-116, 1989.
47. Abe Y, Sakae S, Yamasita T, et al: Vascular hyperpermeability induced by tumor necrosis factor and its augmentation by Il-1 and IFN-γ is inhibited by selective depletion of neutrophils with a monoclonal antibody. J Immunol 145:2902-2907, 1990.
48. Yonemaru M, Hatherill JR, Hoffman H, et al: Pentoxifylline does not attenuate acute lung injury in the absence of granulocytes. J Appl Physiol 71:342-351, 1992.
49. Mier JW, Vachino G, Klempner MS, et al: Inhibition of interleukin-2 induced tumor necrosis factor release by dexamethasone: Prevention of an acquired neutrophil chemotaxis defect and differential suppression of interleukin-2 associated side effect. Blood 76:1933-1940, 1990.
50. Snydman DR, Sullivan B, Gill M, et al: Nosocomial sepsis associated with interleukin-2. Ann Intern Med 112:102-107, 1990.
51. Klempner MS, Noring R, Mier JW, et al: An acquired chemotactic defect in neutrophils from patients receiving interleukin-2 immunotherapy. N Engl J Med 322:959-965, 1990.
52. Jablons D, Bolton E, Mertins S, et al: Il-2-based immunotherapy alters circulating neutrophil Fc receptor expression and chemotaxis. J Immunol 144:3630-3636, 1990.
53. Thijs LB, Hack CE, Strack Van Schijndel JMS, et al: Activation of the complement system during immunotherapy with recombinant Il-2. Relation to the development of side effects. J Immunol 144:2419-2424, 1990.
54. Sagone AL, Husney RM, Triozzi PL, et al: Interleukin-2 therapy enhances salicylate oxidation by blood granulocytes. Blood 78:2931-2936, 1991.
55. Heslop HE, Price GM, Prentice HG, et al: In vitro analysis of the interactions of recombinant Il-2 with regenerating lymphoid and

myeloid cells after allogeneic marrow transplantation. J Immunol 140:3461-3466, 1988.

56. Pober JS, Gimbrone MA, Lapierre LA, et al: Overlapping patterns of activation of human endothelial cells by IL-1, TNF and immune interferon. J Immunol 137:1893-1899, 1986.

57. Puri RK, Rosenberg SA: Combined effects of interferon α and interleukin 2 on the induction of a vascular leak syndrome in mice. Cancer Immunol Immunother 28:267-274, 1989.

58. Kitayama J, Takeo J, Atomi Y, et al: Transendothelial migration activity of lymphokine-activated killer (LAK) cells. J Immunol 151:1663-1672, 1993.

59. Ettinghausen SE, Moore JG, White DE, et al: Hematologic effects of immunotherapy with lymphokine-activated killer cells and recombinant Il-2 in cancer patients. Blood 69:1654-1660, 1987.

60. Aronson FR, Libby P, Brandon EP, et al: Il-2 rapidly induces natural killer cell adhesion to human endothelial cells. A potential mechanism for endothelial injury. J Immunol 141:158- 163, 1988.

61. Damle NK, Doyle LV: IL-2 activated human killer lymphocytes but not their secreted products mediate increase in albumin flux across cutured endothelial monolayer. Implications for vascular leak syndrome. J Immunol 142:2660-2669, 1989.

62. McMannis JD, Fisher RI, Creekmore SP, et al: In vivo effect of recombinant Il-2 I. Isolation of circulating Leu-19+ lymphokine-activated killer effector cells from cancer patients receiving recombinant Il-2. J Immunol 140:1335-1340, 1988.

63. Urba WJ, Steis RG, Longo DL, et al: Immunomodulatory properties and toxicity of interleukin 2 in patients with cancer. Cancer Res 50:185-192, 1990.

64. Abraham VS, Sachs DH, Sykes M: Mechanism of protection from graft-versus-host disease mortality by IL-2. III. Early reactions in donor T cell subsets and expansion of a CD3+CD4+CD8-cell population. J Immunol 148:3746-3752, 1992.

65. Sykes M, Abraham VS, Harty MW, et al: Il-2 reduces graft- versus-host disease and preserves a graft-versus-leukemia effect by selectively inhibiting CD4+ T cell activity. J Immunol 150:197-205, 1993.

66. Goldstein D, Sosman JA, Hank G, et al: Repetitive weekly cycles of Il 2: Effect of outpatient treatment with a lower dose of Il-2 on non-major histocompatibility complex-restricted killer activity. Cancer Res 49:6832-6838, 1989.

67. Blaise D, Olive D, Stoppa AM, et al: Hematolgic and immunologic effects of the systemic administration of recombinant in-

terleukin-2 after autologous bone marrow transplantation. Blood 76:1092-1097, 1990.

68. Weisdorf DJ, Anderson PM, Blazar BR, et al: Interleukin 2 immediately after autologous bone marrow transplantation for acute lymphoblastic leukemia-a phase I study. Transplantation 55:61-66, 1993.

69. Higuchi CM, Thompson JA, Petersen FB, et al: Toxicity and immunomodulatory effects of interleukin-2 after autologous bone marrow transplantation for hematologic malignancies. Blood 77:2561-2568, 1991.

70. Soiffer RJ, Murray C, Cochran K, et al: Clinical and immunologic effects of prolonged infusion of low-dose recombinant interleukin-2 after autologous and T-cell depleted allogeneic bone marrow transplantation. Blood 79:517-526, 1992.

71. Negrier S, Ranchere JY, Philip I, et al: Intravenous interleukin-2 after high dose BCNU and autologous bone marrow transplantation. Report of a multicentric French pilot study. Bone Marrow Transplant 8:259-264, 1991.

72. Hamon MD, Prentice HG, Gottlieb DJ, et al: Immunotherapy with interleukin 2 after ABMT in AML. Bone Marrow Transplant 11:399-401, 1993.

73. Schecter D, Nagler A, Ackerstein A, et al: Recombinant interleukin-2 and interferon alpha immunotherapy following ABMT. A case report of cardiovascular toxicity with serial echocardiographic evaluation. Cardiology 80:168-171, 1992.

74. Malkovsky M, Brenner M, Hunt R, et al: T cell depletion of allogeneic bone marrow prevents acceleration of graft-versus-host disease induced by exogenous Il-2. Cell Immunol 103:476-480, 1986.

75. Benyunes MC, Massumoto C, York A, et al: Interleukin-2 with or without lymphokine-activated killer cells as consolidative immunotherapy after autologous bone marrow transplantation for acute myelogenous leukemia. Bone Marrow Transplant 12:159-163, 1993.

76. Favrot MC, Floret D, Negrier S, et al: Systemic interleukin-2 therapy in children with progressive neuroblastoma after high dose chemotherapy and BMT. Bone Marrow Transplant 4:499-503, 1989.

77. Duncombe AS, Grundy JE, Prentice HG, et al: Il-2 activated killer cells may contribute to cytomegalovirus induced marrow hypoplasia after bone marrow transplantation. Bone Marrow Transplant 7:81-87, 1991.

78. Rosenberg SA, Lotze MT, Muul LM, et al: A progress report on the treatment of 157 patients with advanced cancer using lym-

phokine-activated killer cells and interleukin-2 or high-dose in-terluekin-2 alone. N Engl J Med 316:889-897, 1987.

79. West WH, Tauer KW, Yanelli JR, et al: Constant-infusion recombinant interleukin-2 in adoptive immunotherapy of advanced cancer. N Engl J Med 316:898-905, 1987.
80. Webb DE, Austin HA, Belldegrun A, et al: Metabolic and renal effects of interleukin-2 immunotherapy for metastatic cancer. Clin Nephrol 30:141-145, 1988.
81. Lee RE, Lotze MT, Skibber JM, et al: Cardiorespiratory effects of immunotherapy with interleukin-2. J Clin Oncol 7:7-20, 1989.
82. Belldegrun A, Webb DE, Austin HA, et al. Effects of Il-2 on renal function in patients receiving immunotherapy for advanced cancer. Ann Intern Med 106:817-822, 1987.
83. Papa MZ, Vetto JT, Ettinghausen SE, et al: Effect of corticosteroid on the antitumor activity of lymphokine-activated killer cells and interleukin 2 in mice. Cancer Res 46:5618-5623, 1986.
84. Vetto JT, Papa MZ, Lotze MT, et al: Reduction of toxicity of Il-2 and lymphokine-activated killer cells in humans by administration of corticosteroids. J Clin Oncol 5:496-503, 1987.
85. Manoogain C, Nadler J, Ehrlich L, et al: The renal vasodilating effect of dopamine is mediated by calcium flux and prostacyclin release in man. J Clin Endocrinol Metab 66:678-683, 1988.
86. Yamazaki M, Matsuoka T, Yasui K, et al: Dopamine inhibition of superoxide anion production by polymorphonuclear leukocytes. J Allergy Clin Immunol 83:967-972, 1989.
87. Myers BD, Moran SM: Mechanisms of disease. Hemodynamically mediated acute renal failure. N Engl J Med 314:97-105, 1986.
88. Sinzinger H, Cromwell M, Firbas W: Long-lasting depression of rabbit aortic prostacylcin formation by single-dose irradiation. Radiat Res 97:533-534, 1984.

Index

171